W9-BKB-421

# The Real You Diet

# The Real You Diet

## Your Personal Program for Lasting Weight Loss

Madelyn Fernstrom, Ph.D., CNS

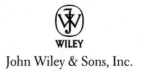

**WILEY**

John Wiley & Sons, Inc.

Published by John Wiley & Sons, Inc., Hoboken, New Jersey
Published simultaneously in Canada

For general information about our other products and services, please contact our Customer Care Department within the United States at (800) 762-2974, outside the United States at (317) 572-3993 or fax (317) 572-4002.

Wiley also publishes its books in a variety of electronic formats. Some content that appears in print may not be available in electronic books. For more information about Wiley products, visit our web site at www.wiley.com.

*Library of Congress Cataloging-in-Publication Data:*
Fernstrom, Madelyn H.
  The real you diet : your personal program for lasting weight loss / Madelyn Fernstrom.
     p. cm.
  Includes index.
  ISBN 978-0-470-37180-0 (cloth) 1. Weight loss—Popular works. 2. Reducing diets—Popular works. 3. Nutrition—Popular works. 4. Physical fitness—Popular works. I. Title.
  RM222.2.F4275 2009
  613.2'5—dc22

                                                                    2009014012

Printed in the United States of America

10  9  8  7  6  5  4  3  2  1

To John, Lauren, and Aaron

# Contents

# Acknowledgments

I am most grateful to my husband and colleague, John D. Fernstrom, Ph.D., who has been a valuable scientific resource and a great support to me. Whether he was answering a question on brain chemistry or taste-testing a recipe, he was always ready to lend a hand (or his taste buds).

Many thanks to my children, Lauren and Aaron, for their constant support and encouragement, as well as their many helpful suggestions.

Never too busy to chat, Alice Martell, my literary agent, was a fountain of positive energy and good ideas, for which I am most appreciative.

Special thanks to Christel Winkler, my editor at Wiley, whose good humor was infectious and whose editorial skills are simply awesome. I am also grateful to Tom Miller for his initial interest and enthusiasm about the book. Rachel Meyers, production editor extraordinaire, provided many insightful suggestions.

I continue to be thankful for my extended family, friends, and patients, who have encouraged me, over the past few years, to write a book like this one in the hopes that it would help others achieve the long-term weight loss success that they did.

# How to Use This Book
## Finding the Real You

**How many times** have you been told you'd lose weight if you just followed "the plan"? And how many times has the burst of enthusiasm brought by your short-term success turned into disappointment? Many times, I think, leading you to consider it your own personal failure. If you had only stuck to the plan, you would have achieved your desired results. That's where the Real You Diet and its BEAM Box approach are different. You don't adapt to the plan, the plan adapts to *you*.

I've spent more than twenty-five years in the clinic and in the laboratory helping people lose weight and keep it off. I know it's not easy. One thing I've learned is that when it comes to weight loss, one size certainly does not fit all. Just as the path to weight gain was different for each of us, so weight loss will require its own individualized approach. I want to help you develop your own, unique way to achieve weight-loss success by choosing tools that work for you (though they may not work for someone else). Finding the right combination of tools right now will also help you maintain your weight over the long haul.

*The Real You Diet* is your new beginning. With some honest self-evaluation, you'll be able to explore and compare all of the comprehensive options for weight loss in one book. This book is your introduction to the four major categories—<u>B</u>ehavioral, <u>E</u>ating, <u>A</u>ctivity, and <u>M</u>edical/biological—that you must consider, as a unit, for effective weight loss and long-term maintenance. These categories will form the foundation of your BEAM Box and set you on the path to lifelong success. While they will provide a solid basis for your weight-loss efforts, you might also need to consider the power tools of medication or surgery to support (but never replace) your lifestyle effort.

There is no right or wrong way to read this book. It provides a comprehensive set of effective tools to get you started in each area. The goal is to continue to build your BEAM Box, using this book and adding your own resources to the mix. I'm hoping the mind-set of *The Real You Diet*, of using the right tool for the right job, will allow you to see the weight-management puzzle in a whole new light and give you confidence. You'll add and take away tools as needed. When you're bored with your plan, you'll replace some worn-out tools with some new, more effective ones.

*The Real You Diet* is your personal road to permanent weight control. It's time you were fully equipped with the right tools for this difficult journey. This time, you are up to the challenge and will succeed, because you'll have the full range of comprehensive tools from which to choose. You are guided along the weight-loss path, with specific choices to make that will let you add your own personal touch.

You're not alone in this journey. Think of me as watching over your shoulder, guiding you along the way. Believe in yourself. When you finally get the right combination of tools in your own BEAM Box, the *real you* will emerge and achieve long-term weight-loss success.

# 1

# The Real You Approach to Weight Loss

**Losing weight is hard.** If it were easy, everyone would be thin. No one wants to carry extra pounds—and it's not for lack of trying that so many of us do. So what's the problem?

For too long we have heard, "Follow this plan, eat this, exercise like that, and you too will lose weight." Taking this approach to its likely conclusion, if a diet doesn't work, it's *our* fault—not the plan's fault. We must be doing something wrong, or else we'd be losing weight. This is a negative approach, which only fuels the basic insecurity we all have about our ability to lose weight and keep it off. We get discouraged and feel that whatever we're doing just isn't working. We go into a downward spiral, get down on ourselves, get discouraged, and give up. Sound familiar?

The old "just push yourself away from the table and run around the block" advice doesn't cut it anymore—and maybe it never did. Here's why I think such a simplistic approach doesn't work. Life is complicated, and it's not a perfect world. We're so busy and stressed, we become disconnected from our body's signals. Much of the time we're just not listening, or we're getting mixed signals, which only diminishes our ability to maintain an effective weight-loss plan.

Everyone reading this book knows that losing weight and keeping it off is a tough challenge. My life's work has been helping people accomplish just this feat. I want to answer the challenge every person poses: "Don't tell me what to do, tell me how to do it!"

When it comes to weight loss, one size does not fit all. Most diet plans are not tailor-made, and that's why so many of them fail. *You* must fit into the plan, and not the other way around. The Real You plan *is* tailor-made. It has an individualized approach, and you put together the tools for a successful weight-loss plan that you can live with comfortably.

To achieve *successful* weight loss and maintenance, you need a complete and comprehensive toolbox. Many of us have some of the tools we need, but not all of them. We haven't spent the time to figure out what's missing.

The Real You plan shows you how to find "the right tool for the right job," as the old saying goes. Or in this case, the right tools for the right person—yourself! You need the right tools to evaluate and address your behavior, eating, activity, and medical (BEAM) issues. That's why I call this personal toolbox a BEAM Box. The Real You plan will help you pick a selection of tools for your personal BEAM Box, which you can turn to again and again throughout your life.

Weight loss can be looked at as a giant jigsaw puzzle with many interconnecting pieces. Your pieces are not the same size and shape as anyone else's. Many factors contribute to weight loss and weight gain. These factors include genetic predisposition, physiological and metabolic issues, emotional and behavioral issues, stress management, cultural and psychosocial patterns, environmental issues, brain chemistry, sleep habits, and many more. From one individual to another, these all play a different role in supporting or sabotaging an effective weight-control plan.

In *The Real You Diet*, we'll take a step-by-step approach to identifying the pieces of your individual weight-loss puzzle and transforming these into practical tools for everyday living. As you read about the individual journeys of some of my patients, I hope you will be able to connect with their experiences in building your own BEAM Box, as they have built theirs. It takes time and mental focus, but it is within the grasp of everyone, no matter what your starting point is or how much weight you want to lose. You can also build a BEAM Box for weight stability, or the "just don't gain" approach. That is also weight-loss success.

To build your BEAM Box, you must be totally honest with yourself and be willing to understand both your personal strengths as well as your personal barriers to effective weight management. Know yourself and accept what you're willing and able to do for a healthy weight. You are good working material! Let's check out the tools and start building.

## Choosing the Tools to Build a BEAM Box

There are four major groups you'll need to incorporate into your basic BEAM Box. I consider them the four major points of the Real You plan foundation. Each of these groups has a selection of tools to meet your needs—my version of the right tool for the right job!

Behavioral

Eating

Activity

Medical/Biological

For those of you who may need to explore further options, additional power tools can be added to support (but not replace) the fundamental four. These are medication (pharmacotherapy), obesity surgery, and body contouring.

Your first step is to take an honest and nonjudgmental look at yourself and to ask yourself if an entire tool group is deficient. You may have to dig a little deeper to see what tools are missing within a particular group. Many people have gaps in all four areas. If that's you, there is no reason for panic. It's okay to tackle one at a time. Others might be missing just one or two pieces of the puzzle, and often that's the reason that weight loss is a struggle for them, even when they feel they're doing everything right.

All the right tools must be in place both to achieve long-term weight loss and to sustain the effort to keep it off. Many of my patients first come in saying, "I'm out of control." When I ask them about any tools they've tried before, they frequently respond, "I have no tools. I don't know what to do!" By getting them to take a step back and think about their own past strengths and weaknesses in the weight-loss battle, in a nonjudgmental way, I usually can help them get a pretty good idea of their starting position. Most people find that they have a reasonable starting set of skills.

The struggle comes when we start a plan and then get tired of the plan's routine. Building structure is essential, but things don't always go as planned, which is why we all need a Plan B. It takes at least a few weeks to establish a set of habits. During that time we have to constantly revisit the issue of what we are both willing and able to do. That's where developing *specialized* tools in all four areas is vital for all of us.

Think about the following questions; you'll see that the answers often involve a combination of overlapping tools needed to find a long-term solution.

- What can I do when I'm bored with my eating plan? (Eating, Behavior)
- What about when I'm feeling deprived? (Behavior, Eating)
- How can I plan an activity I can live with *every day*? (Activity, Behavior, Biology)
- How can I handle food sabotage by friends and family? (Behavior, Eating)
- Can I allow an eating indulgence and still maintain control? (Eating, Behavior)
- How can I recognize contentment as an end point? (Medical, Behavior, Eating)
- Can "free foods" take the pressure off mental hunger? (Eating, Behavior)
- Should I talk with my doctor about prescription medications? (Medical, Eating, Activity, Behavior)
- Should I consider a surgical option? (Medical, Eating, Behavior, Activity)
- Can I do something about loose skin after weight loss? (Medical, Activity, Eating, Behavior)

# The Four-Point Foundation of the BEAM Box

While you may be tempted to jump to a particular category of interest, I hope you'll take a look at the next four chapters *before* you start to build your BEAM Box. Or, for a quick overview, take a look at the list of tools in appendix C. It's a good way to take an inventory of your needs before beginning the plan.

## 1. Behavioral Tools

When I think of behavioral change, I think of the willingness to try new things and about the lifestyle issues of eating, exercising, and stress management in a new way. I also think about individual temperaments. Some people are naturally optimistic and are the "glass half-full" thinkers. Some of us are the "glass half-empty" thinkers, expecting things to go wrong. Most people are somewhere in-between and can swing between both extremes from time to time, particularly when it comes to weight loss.

Think of the beginning of a weight-loss plan. Eternal optimism. A fresh start. You're told precisely what to eat and how to exercise. It *must* work. Since the typical plan is not personally tailored to *you*, but to some imaginary perfect-world person, you usually start out strong, complying with what the diet asks. Then real life intervenes, and the novelty wears off. The natural optimism of the new plan falls by the wayside and a sense of impending doom sets in. What started with a bang ends in another diet failure.

With this plan, you can expect different results. When you take a step back, and first identify—and accept—those behaviors that are sabotaging your efforts to remain *consistent* in a weight-loss plan, incorporating them into your BEAM Box, you can utilize the best set of behavioral strategies that work for you.

What your behavioral tools will provide is realistic optimism. You'll select a starter set of behavioral changes to make, and you'll build on them. When you find you're struggling (which we all do), rather than panic and collapse, you'll be able to tweak your plan, to stay on track, and to learn from your mistakes.

## 2. Eating Tools

Many of my patients laugh when we first start to talk about what to eat. "I'm a walking encyclopedia of food facts," say many. And I believe them. This set of tools is to make food work for *you*. We must all make friends with food, because unlike smoking or drinking, *we have to eat*. Nature provides an inborn drive to eat for survival, and nothing can take that survival signal away. We must learn to manage that biological signal and separate it from all other reasons for eating.

Here is where I ask you to take an honest look at your food likes and dislikes. We are often confused by what foods are considered "healthy" or pressured to consume the "right" foods for weight loss, without ever taking into account food composition, taste, texture, and enjoyment. Enjoyment and eating? Do those two actually go together? Of course! *Food* choice, not just nutrient and calorie choice, is what we're looking at here. We all have food preferences and aversions, and you'll learn to personalize your eating plan to match your eating style. My favorite motto is: "There are no bad foods, just bad portions."

Calorie *awareness* is a key tool in this area. It is possible to lose weight with either a protein-focused or a carbohydrate-focused approach. It all depends on the food selection and calorie content. While many research studies compete to show which plan is best, there's really very little evidence that one strategy is better than another. I believe it's hard to interpret the compliance results of many research studies, since participants are rarely given the option of which particular diet plan of the comparison they personally *prefer*, and are simply assigned to a group. That certainly can influence their motivation, focus, and long-term success.

We select foods for many reasons, and the eating tools will help you choose foods and structure your meal plans in order to achieve the nutritional balance that nature intended. You will learn to navigate a world where food is available 24/7. The eating tools will transform you into a mindful eater, to really connect not only with the foods you choose, but with the biological signals for hunger and fullness.

## 3. Activity Tools

*Move more.* Sounds easy, so why is it so hard for most of us? Those two words are a huge barrier for many reasons. How and when you do it are negotiable. What does "moving more" actually mean to most of us? Of the whole toolbox, this is often the area where there's the most confusion about what to do. It all seems too time-consuming and a chore. What is the most frequent reason I hear from patients about their inactivity? "Lack of time." The next most common reason is the lack of confidence that activity can make a difference in a weight-loss plan, unless it's a punishing routine. Confusion abounds about building muscle, developing core strength, and activity's relation to heart health. This tool group will distinguish the different types of physical activity and show you how you can mix and match them to meet your personal needs. You'll want to evaluate the kinds of activities that you enjoy and are comfortable doing. Plus, you'll learn how to make a change when you become bored—and even how to recognize boredom. (Do you really hate the treadmill, or are you just tired of it?)

A key feature here is to separate *mental fatigue* from *physical fatigue*, which are often confused with each other. Both make us feel exhausted. The goal is to move more, no matter what you're doing—it all helps. From the activity of daily living to competitive sports, you will get to choose the combination of tools to mix and match for long-term commitment.

## 4. Medical/Biological Tools

While most people say, "I feel good enough, I just have to lose weight," many have not seen their doctor for quite a while—even those on prescription medications for illnesses often related to weight! Whether you're too busy to make an appointment, or you dread the embarrassment of a skimpy examination gown, or even just getting on the scale, a visit to your doctor is a must-do, to identify what I call "hidden barriers" to weight loss. (These are described in chapter 2.) These can only be determined by a blood test and a physical exam. It's important to rule out—or treat—some biological causes, such as hormone imbalances and certain prescription medications, that can interfere with even the best lifestyle efforts.

## Power Tools: Supporting a Lifestyle Effort

Adding the power tool of medication or surgery is always a tough decision, and the pros and cons should be discussed to determine your own personal risk-to-benefit ratio. At one end of the spectrum, you hear it's a "quick fix" or "the easy way out." This is particularly true when it comes to discussions of weight-loss surgery. Your first step in considering these options is to embrace the idea that a power tool can only support, *but not replace,* your lifestyle effort. This core understanding must be part of any discussion of a power tool. The addition of power tools comes after a thorough evaluation of how the four core sets of tools are working (or not). When it comes to adding power tools successfully, it's all in the right timing.

## Finding the Real You

A final thought before we move on to the important beginning steps of building your new toolbox. The first step is self-evaluation—how to size yourself up before choosing your tools. As you read the next chapter, think about a journey of self-awareness to develop personal insights that fuel success and help explain past sabotage. No matter what size package you are in right now, you'll be able to pack your BEAM Box with everything you need if you listen to the most important person of all: *you.*

# 2

# Size Yourself Up
## How to Create Your BEAM Box

**The Real You plan** is based on knowing what you are both willing and able to do to sustain a long-term commitment to weight control. That's what building a BEAM Box is all about. Your personal toolbox will be selected from the four-point BEAM foundation, with all points equally essential for real-life weight control. In the four chapters that follow this one, I'll lay out these tools for you to pick and choose what feels right for you. Don't expect your combination of tools to be identical to those of your friends, or even of your closest loved ones. You want to find the perfect fit to meet your needs both for now and for the future, when (not if!) you need a change in your plan. Only a personally tailored plan that meets your own needs will give you the confidence and commitment needed to lose weight and keep it off.

## Ten Steps to Building Your BEAM Box

It all starts with baby steps. I've laid out ten basic steps to get you started on building your BEAM Box.

While I suggest a few general time guidelines in some of the steps, there's no rush or pressure to get through any of them. Many people can complete the ten steps in six to eight weeks, but I want you to rely on your internal timer. Some steps you'll breeze right through, and others may take more time. What's most important is following each step *until* you feel confident that you've mastered it, and *only then* moving on to the next one.

1. **Discover the real you.** Evaluate yourself by taking all four mini-quizzes in this chapter. Your score will determine what tools you will need and where you need to focus particular effort. Everyone is unique and has a different starting point. You might already have the right tools in one area but need more help with another. You may want a fresh start and need to build a foundation from the ground up.

2. **Visit your doctor.** If you haven't seen your primary care doctor (or gynecologist) in the past six months, schedule a visit. No primary care doctor? Talk with your friends and family to find one. Check with your insurance company for a complete listing of physicians in your network.

3. **Upgrade your equipment.** Purchase a simple pedometer (no talking, calories, or strides required) that just counts steps. Accusplit (www.accusplit.com) is one that meets my three criteria for a pedometer: it's economical, easy to use, and accurate. If you want to invest more money, go ahead and select a more elaborate model, but it's not a must-have to track your activity. The most important thing is to wear it every day.

   Get a reliable home scale. You'll want a digital model, one that is economical and only indicates weight. No need to spend extra (unless you want to) for body fat, muscle mass, or other measures that don't change quickly. These add on a lot of cost, for marginal return. If your scale records all different weights depending on where you have it placed in your bathroom, or you're squinting to look at a needle on a nondigital scale, it's definitely time for a new scale.

4. **Pick the tools for your BEAM Box.** Review all the tools described in each of the four BEAM chapters (or consult the quick list in appendix C) and pick some tools from each group that immediately interest you. Write them down, and review them daily. Scan the list for those that jump out at you as tools you are both willing and able to try. It's also worthwhile to take a look at the Fernstrom Fundamentals to stay connected for daily inspiration. They are listed briefly at the end of this chapter and explained in more depth in chapter 3.

5. **Get started!** Chapter 7 lays out a twenty-one-day plan with activity goals and meal plans. A starting to-do list will help you call upon all four points of your BEAM Box foundation. Here is where you will begin to put your tools to work for you.

   The first seven days of the Real You plan are meant to help you form new habits, and the next fourteen days are geared toward sustaining those habits. As you implement the twenty-one days of your Real You eating plan, you will begin to discover which tools are working for you and which ones you might want to change.

6. **Form new habits.** Evaluate your first seven days on the plan. If you feel you can maintain the changes you've made and you like your lifestyle selections, then don't change anything. Stick with what you have and see if you can maintain these healthy changes for another two weeks. You can get more eating ideas from the next fourteen days of meal plans or simply continue with your choices from the first seven days. That's three weeks with your BEAM Box—the time it takes to form a new set of habits. Review chapters 3, 4, 5, and 6 to reinforce and expand your plan.

7. **Sticking to it.** If you have not lost at least 3 pounds by the end of three weeks, don't panic. Take the quizzes in this chapter again. See if there are any areas where you feel vulnerable, and choose more tools from that specific area. Do a little "reverse calorie counting" (see chapter 4) and trim 200 calories per day from your

current eating plan. Keep wearing your pedometer, and aim to increase your total steps by 1,000 every day. Haven't yet made an appointment with your doctor, or still haven't found one? Do it now. You may be facing some unknown medical/biological issues that are sabotaging even your best efforts.

8. **Keep things interesting.** Start bartering and exchanging within the food categories to avoid getting bored or disengaged while staying consistent in your calorie intake (see chapter 4). If you're still happy with your original plan, there's no need to change until you feel like it.

9. **Stay active.** Review your physical activity plan. Make sure you are maintaining thirty minutes of "daily living activities." Aim to add a planned aerobic/cardio activity or strength training (see chapter 5) at least once a week if you haven't already done so.

10. **Evaluate your success.** Take a look at the rate of weight loss you have achieved from using your present BEAM Box. If you haven't lost at least 5 pounds in the past six weeks, talk to your health provider about possible biological hidden causes of weight gain (see chapter 6).

    Evaluate whether your lifestyle log has been converted to your "mental database." That's the point where you feel you've mastered the foundation of your lifestyle and you no longer need to keep a daily written log.

## Maintain and Sustain for Life

*Your new eating and activity plan is now a lifestyle.* You've mentally ingrained your own BEAM Box, and your responses are automatic. From this time on, revisit your BEAM Box every two weeks. Make sure you weigh yourself at least once a week, but not more often than once a day. Check to make sure you are not bored with your food choices and are maintaining structure. Make sure your activity level is consistent and you're getting at least thirty minutes of daily living activity, with vigorous activity two or more times a week. ("Vigorous" means you're using enough energy that you can't talk while doing the activity.)

At the end of eight weeks, or whatever time period you feel comfortable with, you should be reasonably confident that your BEAM Box is filled with the essential tools that work for you. While you can add and switch tools in all categories, you've done the hard work to establish the foundation of good health. You have your "workhorse" tools for every day, and then the tools you pull out now and then. When you feel stalled, or need a change, go back to "boot camp," where you can revisit and adapt your BEAM Box to reflect your current needs.

## When to Consider Using Power Tools

While your BEAM Box is the foundation of your healthy lifestyle plan, you may need to think about adding the power tools of prescription medication and/or surgery to support your lifestyle effort. Your first step must always be to accept that these power tools can support, but not replace, the lifestyle effort. Medication and surgery may be the missing tools for your BEAM Box.

**Months 3 to 6:** Interested in prescription medications? Review chapter 8 to see if you meet the medical criteria for medications, and if the action of these medicines meets both your medical needs and your eating style. A visit to your doctor will help you evaluate this next step. (*Important note:* If you are not a candidate for medication, and your body mass index [BMI] is 40 or over, you can go directly to considering a surgical option for more help. Check out appendix A to learn how to calculate your BMI.)

**Months 6 to 12:** If you've tried a medication and it is not a good support to your lifestyle, you might want to consider obesity surgery. Review chapter 8 to see if you meet the surgical criteria. Start with a visit to your primary care doctor to discuss this option, and get a referral to a Center of Excellence Surgical Program.

# The Self-Evaluation Process

It's now time to take a fresh, honest look at yourself, eyes wide open—no squinting—to find the real you. Here's where you evaluate your personal strengths and weaknesses. While we all have strengths we can rattle off when it comes to weight loss, it's the personal barriers we face that sabotage our lifestyle effort and get us down and discouraged. No one is a perfect eater or exerciser. We all get stressed-out, go off track, and struggle. There is always room for improvement. While it's important to feel good about the positive changes we make, it's equally essential to tackle our barriers to success. *Honestly* sizing yourself up helps you to better start selecting your first set of tools. Chapter 1 explained the four kinds of tools you'll need to build your BEAM Box. Now it's time to take the first step and do a self-evaluation of your starting point.

For some of you, this task is easy, a no-brainer. For others, it takes some time and effort to tease out the essential, and missing, tools. With that in mind, I'd like you to take four mini-quizzes to identify your vulnerable areas in each of the BEAM categories. Don't worry if you need help in all four of them. Most of us do. The number of tools you begin with is unimportant, it's just getting started that counts. These are tools for life, and in the process of building your complete BEAM Box, you'll continue to add tools at your own pace.

In each of the quizzes that follow, answer the questions with a yes or no. Add up your yes replies.

### Your Behavioral Awareness

1. Do you eat when you're stressed?
2. Do you sneak food when no one is looking?
3. Do you feel guilty when you eat dessert?
4. Do you eat when you're bored?
5. Do you eat first, and think about your food choices later?
6. Do you sleep less than six hours a night?
7. Do you eat even when you feel physically satisfied?
8. Do you eat more when you're happy?

If you answered yes to four or more questions, then your behavioral tools are missing or rusty. Check out chapter 3 for more help. You'll be able to select a variety of tools that provide support and solutions in areas where you need it the most.

## Your Eating Awareness

1. Do you jump from plan to plan to lose weight?
2. Do you easily get bored with an eating plan?
3. Are you confused about the basics of healthy eating?
4. Do you skip reading food labels?
5. Do you eat whenever food is around you?
6. Do you think you don't drink enough fluid during the day?
7. Do you count everything except calories?
8. Do you skip meals?

If you answered yes to four or more questions, your eating tools need some help. In chapter 4 you will learn to make food work for you rather than against you.

## Your Activity Awareness

1. Do you feel you are too busy to exercise?
2. Did you used to be more active than you are now?
3. Do you ignore the urge to move when it strikes?
4. Do you save your physical activity for the weekends?
5. Do you think exercise counts less than eating to lose weight?
6. Do you have physical limitations for exercise?
7. Do you feel overwhelmed by the idea of daily exercise?
8. Are you confused about the "best" exercise options?

If you answered yes to four or more questions, you need to give special attention to your physical activity needs discussed in chapter 5. Here you'll learn how to add more activity to your daily life in ways that are compatible with your interests and exercise temperament.

## Your Medical Awareness

1. Are you embarrassed to go to your doctor?
2. Do you avoid discussing your weight issues with your doctor?
3. Do you have medical illnesses related to your weight?
4. Do you take prescription medications for your medical illnesses?

5. Have you ever been told you have metabolic syndrome?
6. Do you think medicine you take contributes to your weight gain?
7. Are you unsure of your height and weight?
8. Do you think your body is fighting your weight-loss efforts?

If you answered yes to four or more questions, your medical tools need some work. Chapter 6 will tell you how to have an honest and effective discussion with your doctor about your weight.

# Hidden Causes of Weight Gain

I'd like you to think about the hidden causes of weight gain. This is particularly important for those who feel they've tried everything to lose weight and it's still not coming off. It's a critical step to understanding important tools you might consider.

If you've been struggling with your weight for what seems a lifetime (or actually may be), check out the hidden causes described below and see how fixable they can be, once you have identified them and built the right tools around them. How do these examples apply to you?

### Hidden Behavioral Causes of Weight Gain

**Lack of sleep.** Not enough sleep is among the top hidden reasons for weight struggles. With fatigue, many people eat for energy. Being tired leads to lack of focus and to "not caring" about a lifestyle plan. People fall back on between-meal snacking to wake up, when a power nap is really what's needed.

**Poor stress management.** Mindless eating comes from lack of focus, and poor coping skills with the stressors in our lives. We eat to soothe ourselves, or to reward ourselves, and we indulge in extra calories—which does work, temporarily—to make us feel better. It's important to learn to self-soothe and manage stress responses without food.

**Lack of consistency.** Some general awareness every day is needed to avoid what I call "weight creep." It takes only 100 calories extra a day to gain 10 pounds in a year. Most often, people "relax" their lifestyle on the weekend, or stay on their plan four or five days a week. That's enough to promote a pound or two a month of hidden weight gain.

## Hidden Eating Causes of Weight Gain

**Confusing "heart-healthy" or "fat-free" with low-calorie.** Reading a food label these days is like reading an encyclopedia; so much information is given, but what really counts? There is a huge amount of confusion about "healthy" versus "lower-calorie" eating. While the first step in any healthy eating plan is to seek out heart-healthy fat, don't be fooled by product marketing. "Healthy" claims on food packaging don't automatically translate to calorie savings. Olive oil is great for your heart, but not for your waistline; both olive oil and butter (artery-clogging fat) have the same calories. Nuts are heart-healthy and protein rich—but just a small handful has 100 calories! Trans fat–free doesn't mean fat-free. Nowadays it's all about reading labels to avoid falling into this confusing trap of health versus calories.

**Portion distortion.** None of us is very good at eyeballing portion sizes or at estimating the calories in foods. Studies show we're at least 50 percent too low in our "guesstimates," even professionals in the field. While we feel we're doing a reasonable job, the cues to do so—plate size, utensil size, hidden fats, and more—all set us up for failure. In fact, the average dinner plate in Europe is close to what we use for a salad plate. Our dinner plates are like platters. No wonder standard portions look skimpy! We've got to learn to downsize our portions.

**Skipping meals.** Whether it's to save time or calories, most meal skippers don't pay attention here and don't think it matters. The most frequent line I hear is: "I skip meals, but it's not a problem until I get home for dinner. Then, I'm eating all night." Here's the bottom line: if we skip a meal, biology kicks in and makes us overly hungry for the next meal. This strategy is doomed to fail.

## Hidden Activity Causes of Weight Gain

**Too much exercise.** How could this backfire? Rigorous exercise actually stimulates hunger. It's the body's response to refuel for metabolic balance. In caveman times, this was helpful for survival, but not now, when food is available 24/7 and we are not foraging in the wilderness for food. We can sometimes fool ourselves into thinking our body needs more calories than it does for weight-stable refueling.

**Overestimating exercise calories burned.** As with food, we don't estimate the calories we've used in exercise very well. We might feel sweaty and think we've burned thousands of calories, based on time spent exercising, but it's best to really know the distance covered. It can take about five minutes to consume 500 calories and nearly two hours for most people to burn it off!

**No exercise.** Those claiming they are simply too busy for any activity can have a real problem. Even a small drop in daily activity—cutting out a twenty-minute walk each day—can add 100 calories a day and 10 pounds in a year. Here's a perfect example: "I used to park blocks away in a cheaper parking lot. I was promoted, and got a spot in the corporate lot. I've gained five pounds in three months." Small activity changes make a difference.

## Hidden Medical Causes of Weight Gain

**Medications.** Some medications can lower the body's metabolic rate and stimulate hunger as a side effect. These include some antidepressants, antipsychotic medicines, antihistamines, insulin and other blood sugar regulators, and anti-inflammatory medicines. If you've started a *new* medicine and gained 4 pounds or more in a month, this might be a contributor. If you've gained weight after months or years on the same medication, it's unlikely that the medication in question is the cause.

**Undiagnosed mood disorders.** Depression and anxiety have both biological and behavioral causes. While some people struggling with depression express symptoms including loss of appetite, insomnia, and weight loss, a large subgroup sleeps more, eats more, and gains weight. Plus, thyroid problems, which can alter weight, are often linked to depression.

**Thyroid function.** The thyroid gland is your body's "furnace" and sets your thermostat. It is regulated by a signal from the brain to release thyroid hormone into the system, and alterations in this gland can wreak havoc on a weight-management plan. The thyroid is easily tested and treated with a visit to your doctor. There are many causes of thyroid problems, and only a visit to your doctor and a blood test can diagnose them.

**Elevated blood insulin.** Also known as "insulin resistance," elevated blood insulin is a main symptom of a medical condition known as "metabolic syndrome." It's invisible unless you get a blood measurement. The constellation of symptoms that occur with metabolic syndrome includes not only high insulin levels, but central weight gain (belly fat), elevated blood pressure, and high cholesterol. Those with an "apple" shape can be at particular risk. Only your doctor can evaluate this important medical issue.

## Fernstrom Fundamentals: Twelve Steps to Long-Term Weight-Loss Success

Let's turn for a minute to some other areas of self-awareness and goal-setting. I've taken some of the basic tools and distilled them into an easy set of fundamentals upon which a strong basis for success is established. These are twelve concepts you must embrace for your toolbox to serve you well. Check out chapter 3 for the specifics of how to use this practical set of tools. These fundamentals are at the foundation of all successful BEAM Boxes.

I've outlined the basic areas and concepts for you to integrate into your own plan. You should be able to use these to identify previous barriers to weight-loss success and help you think about realistic goal setting.

**Fernstrom Fundamentals**

1. Stay connected.
2. Think before you eat anything.
3. Recognize contentment. Look for Level 2 of fullness.
4. Minimize mindless eating.
5. Agree that there are no bad foods, just bad portions.
6. Learn to barter.
7. Keep your mouth busy with noncalorie items.
8. Buy single servings.
9. Accept your temperament.
10. Remind yourself that daily physical activity is important.
11. Wear a pedometer.
12. Don't beat yourself up. Learn from your mistakes.

Now, with the first tool of self-awareness, and understanding of your strengths and weaknesses under your belt, let's take a step-by-step look at how to build your own BEAM Box. Thoroughly read the next four chapters, which describe in detail the tools for each of the four core points of your foundation. In building your BEAM Box, the more tools you understand, the more you will be able to use.

If you are eager to get started right away with an eating plan, you can go directly to chapter 7. There you will find a three-week plan to get you started with structured meals and menu plans, along with some activity guidelines. You might prefer to jump-start your process; just be sure to review all the tools while you are doing it. A list of menus and recipes is not enough without incorporating the tools you need to succeed. The best way to maximize your resources and optimize your success on your weight-loss journey is to build an effective BEAM Box to aid you along the way.

# 3

# Behavioral Tools
## Breaking Those Barriers to Success

"I know what to do to lose weight, but I just can't seem to do it." Sound familiar? The hard fact to accept is that when it comes to losing weight, being willing and being able are not the same thing. "Should I choose the apple or the apple pie?" Some contest! The million-dollar (pound?) questions are: Why can't we choose the apple over the apple pie for better weight control? Why do we go to the movies after a big dinner and buy popcorn and candy? The concept behind the Real You plan can be boiled down to recognizing the kind of changes you are both willing *and* able to make to improve your lifestyle.

You might tell me, "I'm willing to do *anything* to lose weight." But when we scratch the surface, we discover that being willing is not really enough. That's why it's also important to look at what you're *able* to do. Let's take a look at the kinds of problems you need to address, and consider how some behavioral tools can have a real impact on your ability to lose weight and keep it off.

# The Ten Most Important Behavioral Tools

## 1. Work with Your Eating Style

Your personal eating style is a reflection of your individual preferences that you alone determine. It's a matter of what naturally appeals to you in two concrete areas: (1) the flavor and texture of particular foods, and (2) the times of day and how often you prefer to eat. When you can accept your personal eating style, you'll be able to develop some good behavioral tools to match what feels natural to you. You can play to your existing strengths and maximize your behavioral changes. Use your combination of preferences to select the best tools for an eating pattern you can live with for the long term.

Your goal in this section is to identify the kinds of eating patterns you naturally gravitate toward and then tailor your eating to work with, not against, your natural habits. Trust me, it works! Here's a list of some key factors necessary to identify your own eating style. Choose from among the options on this checklist to describe you. Do you recognize yourself here?

Are you:

| _____ a grazer | or | _____ a three-meal-a-day eater? |
|---|---|---|
| _____ a protein lover | or | _____ a carb lover? |
| _____ a day eater | or | _____ a night eater? |
| _____ a home cook | or | _____ a restaurant eater? |
| _____ a intense taster | or | _____ a volume eater? |

**Grazer versus Three-Meal-a-Day Eater**   A grazer enjoys eating many times throughout the day. The concept of mini-meals appeals to the grazer, who achieves a sense of control without deprivation by having a constant stream of calories, in small amounts, seven to eight or more times a day.

_Pros:_ Eating frequently provides a continuing sense of satisfaction.

_Cons:_ Calorie control can be a problem with such frequent eating.

The three-meal-a-day eater likes a routine that is easy and convenient, with a manageable structure and without a major time commitment.

Monitoring calories is easier, since food is consumed fewer times a day, even when you include an optional snack. It's important to allow for one snack a day to avoid possible between-meal hunger.

> *Pros:* Calorie and nutrient monitoring is easier; structure is provided without rigidity.
>
> *Cons:* You can risk becoming over-hungry, especially on days of greater activity. It's important to be mindful of your sense of contentment, and add one snack a day if needed to avoid between-meal hunger.

**Protein Lover versus Carb Lover**   The protein lover enjoys a variety of concentrated proteins—such as chicken, fish, lean beef, and their by-products, including eggs and low-fat dairy. The protein lover is typically not a big fan of vegetable proteins (such as soy and other beans). Protein lovers enjoy eggs and/or yogurt for breakfast and consider protein the basis for most other meals.

> *Pros:* A protein-rich diet provides significant biological satisfaction.
>
> *Cons:* There is a risk of some nutritional deficiencies if carbohydrates are avoided; vegetables and fruits should be the carbohydrates of choice.

The carbohydrate lover prefers starchy carbohydrates as the main eating attraction, with protein as a side dish. Many are also fruit and vegetable lovers, although some prefer starches over fruits and veggies. Vegetable proteins such as soy and other beans are often favored over more concentrated sources.

> *Pros:* Fiber-rich carbohydrates provide volume and fullness. Fruits and vegetables as a main source of carbohydrates provide both fiber and water.
>
> *Cons:* Unless whole grains are selected, calorie excess usually occurs, to give a sense of fullness. Portion distortion can be a problem with calorie-dense starches.

**Day Eater versus Night Eater**   Day eaters prefer to eat most of their daily calories during the day, with the final calories consumed at dinner. The day eater has very little interest in eating in the evening, and has no need for an evening snack.

*Pros:* It's easier to distribute calories throughout the day. The hunger sensation is in place for breakfast, after a period of food deprivation from a good night's sleep.

*Cons:* There are no negatives, other than the risk of getting overly hungry if an active evening is ahead. You should pay attention to hunger and fullness signals.

Night eaters are often busy during the day and do not have much time for or interest in daytime meals and snacks. Night eaters particularly enjoy after-dinner snacking, which they often associate with relaxation and freedom from stress. Night eaters always choose after dinner as the time for their daily snack intervals.

*Pros:* Caloric bartering, and saving 200 calories a day for the evening, provide a lot of satisfaction and contentment.

*Cons:* This style can lead to meal skipping during the day in the hope of saving calories for the evening and then being vulnerable to overeating at night.

**Home Cook versus Restaurant Eater**   The home cook fails to find the appeal of restaurant eating and eats most meals at home. The home cook shops and prepares food regularly and has reasonably tight control of both food ingredients and portion size.

*Pros:* There is no question of hidden fat and calories in self-prepared food. Portions are self-determined. It's a great plan.

*Cons:* It's hard to find a negative here. However, the ability to get a second helping is just steps away, so portion size needs to be monitored.

The restaurant eater is someone who by choice, or as a professional necessity, eats most meals in a restaurant or on the go. We're not talking about the weekend restaurant eater, who enjoys an evening out once a week or less.

*Pros:* There's a lot of variety, which helps you avoid boredom, but you must be an assertive customer to get what you want and maintain a calorie-controlled meal.

*Cons:* There are hundreds of hidden calories from fat in restaurant meals, from fine dining to fast foods. You can't even taste them.

**Intense Taster versus Volume Eater**   The intense taster is someone who prefers a smaller serving of the "real thing" and savors the complexity of taste. The intense taster enjoys full-fat products, a variety of seasonings and spices, and all five of the major taste bud stimulants: sweet, sour, salty, bitter, and umami (savory).

> *Pros:* Smaller portions of food containing original ingredients, including full fats, are satisfying and flavorful.

> *Cons:* Preplanned portion control is key, to avoid consuming too many calories. Eyeballing of portions doesn't work with this approach.

The volume eater doesn't care as much what the food tastes like, as long as it's a large serving. The volume eater is willing to sacrifice some flavor for lower calories and more food. Substitutions to lower fat and sugar and increase fiber content are all part of the volume eater's preferences.

> *Pros:* Eating lower-density foods (fewer calories per serving) is a good way to maintain satisfaction without overconsuming calories.

> *Cons:* There's a risk that all the substitutions provide a final product that lacks flavor, and so you can unwittingly increase portions in search of more flavor.

## 2. Learn to Change a Habit

We all have eating behaviors we'd like to change. You might be surprised to know that creating a new habit takes at least three to four weeks. The first step is the recognition that something has to be changed. That's where a bit of self-reflection always helps. It doesn't just fly out of thin air because you want to make a change. You need to identify a single behavior you want to change, and tackle it one day at a time.

Only when you become aware of your eating patterns are you able to change them. That's why writing down what you eat is an important first step, so any trouble spots become clearer. It's the main reason for keeping your food records. Sometimes it's not so easy to do on your own. You might need a trusted friend, a support group, or a private therapist as an added tool to help you identify your habit and support positive behavior change.

*Ellen's Story*
## I'm Not a Breakfast Eater

It was hard for Ellen to acknowledge that one of her major diet sabotages was skipping breakfast. "I'm just not hungry," she told me. She rationalized her view by saying, "I can save those calories for lunch, when I'm actually hungry." Here's how we changed that habit. Ellen's old view of breakfast was that she had to eat the minute she woke up, still bleary-eyed from sleep. When she changed her idea of breakfast to eating a "morning meal," she saw how this strategy could fit in with her lifestyle. She always stopped at a coffee shop on her way to work for a strong coffee, so she agreed that she would purchase a 20-ounce skim-milk latte instead. She got her morning caffeine (a double shot of espresso), plus 16 ounces of skim milk. This provided a protein boost (16 grams) and a calorie bargain (180 calories). In reality, Ellen was consuming her breakfast at 8:30 a.m. instead of at 7 a.m. She also gained more control over her lunchtime choices because she did not become overly hungry from meal-skipping.

The best part of making this new habit, though, was that it set a structure to her day. Ellen began her day on a positive, healthful note, a reminder that she was connected to her plan at the start of the day. After about six weeks, Ellen expanded her breakfast options to include a 200-calorie protein bar and a large black coffee (she loved her coffeehouse) on days when she felt more like biting into something. This solution was perfect for her.

## 3. Identify Reasons for Emotional Eating

"Emotional eating" is a catch-all term that includes so many things, you've first got to sort out *what kind of emotional eater you are* before you can find the tools to address the particulars. Here are five of the most common triggers for emotional eating. There are many variations on these themes, so see if this helps you identify your own emotional issues with food. When you can identify the problem behavior, you can make a plan to change it that works for you.

## Love of Food

You're a person who loves to shop for food, cook food, and serve food. You derive great pleasure from the taste of food. Often referred to as the "happy eater," you're someone who needs to better manage your portions when consuming the finished product.

If you are a food lover, here are constructive ways to make this emotional trigger work to your benefit:

- Shop for seasonal, locally grown produce to optimize natural flavors.
- Experiment with herbs and spices to intensify flavors, helping to keep you satisfied with smaller portions.
- Downsize your plates and bowls, and get the satisfaction of "eating the whole thing," but in smaller amounts.
- Experiment with making small reductions in added fats, invisible to your family, when preparing your favorite recipes.

### *Stephanie's Story*
## I Love to Cook!

When Stephanie came to see me, she expressed a great sense of sadness over what she thought would be the end of her relationship with cooking and tasty foods in the name of weight loss. A public relations executive by profession, she was a self-described "foodie" and loved to cook. She baked from scratch and had a vast cookbook collection as well as online sources for food-related items ranging from kitchen tools to exotic spices. A favorite regular weekend activity with her husband was dining in new restaurants. At thirty-eight, Stephanie had been experiencing weight creep for the past five years, and she found herself with an extra 40 pounds that just "snuck up" on her. Always at the higher end of healthy BMI (around 24.5), she was now inching toward the higher end of the overweight category, which was a real wakeup call for her. While food was not only her hobby but her passion, she felt that she needed to make a life change in her relationship with food, to both avoid her continuing weight creep and lose some weight. She and her husband planned to start a family "sometime before I turn forty," and she was particularly motivated to lose weight for her general health, as well as in anticipation of a healthy pregnancy.

Stephanie was relieved to hear that she could maintain her close relationship with food, but under a different set of fundamentals. Since she was such a happy eater, she viewed food as a positive force in her life—"A little *too* positive," she said with a laugh—and this positivity formed the basis for her new program. We translated her interest in all things food-related into some specific activities that would help her limit her calories without making her feel deprived: (1) cooking more at home; (2) shopping for high-quality fresh ingredients; (3) choosing locally grown produce; (4) using flavor-intensifying seasonings; (5) modifying the recipes she followed; and (6) concentrating on food presentation.

Stephanie shopped "European style," stopping at a smaller specialty market on her way home from work. She focused more on what was fresh and locally grown in the market, as well as organic produce, dairy, and meats, which she felt offered superior flavor. She also shopped for granular sea salts and peppers from different regions of the world, as well as other spices and seasonings to magnify flavor. Also on her list were highest-quality (and deepest-flavor) olive oils, so she could use less and not compromise on flavor. Stephanie's new adjustment with recipes was to lower the total fat and maintain flavor. She also took an interest in vegetarian cooking and began to use vegetable proteins regularly. She still enjoyed reading all of her cooking and food magazines, but now we agreed that she would use them more to view new trends; plus, she added a subscription to *Cooking Light* magazine for more ideas on recipe substitution. While Stephanie still enjoyed eating in restaurants, she agreed that she would limit this to twice a month and cook for friends at her home on the alternate weekends.

Stephanie also made a commitment to walk for thirty minutes, five days a week, something she felt was manageable for her. For now, that was the limit of her physical activity—what she was both willing and able to do consistently. In her first four weeks, Stephanie lost 5 pounds by sticking with her small but consistent changes. In the next eight weeks, she lost an additional 7 pounds. Losing 12 pounds in three months was energizing for Stephanie, and she expressed relief that she had lost weight without feeling like her "food life" was over. She was firmly in control of a workable plan, with moderate effort and sustained results. A month later, she was down another 3 pounds, the halfway mark to her target, confident that she could continue for the long haul.

---

## Stress

Stress is the classic pitfall of the mindless eater. The hand-to-mouth repetitive activity is soothing. So is the variety of food textures that range from crunchy (a great stress reliever—all that chewing) to smooth and creamy (giving a sense of indulgence). The stress eater needs to replace high-calorie foods with low-calorie items and lots of low-cal beverages. The stress eater is usually a very "oral" person—and needs to keep the mouth busy while consuming fewer calories.

If stress is your emotional trigger to overeat, here are four constructive ways to handle the impulse:

- Chew sugarless gum.
- Crunch on raw vegetables.
- Open bagged salad and eat right from the bag.
- Drink water, seltzer, or a variety of low-calorie water-based drinks.

*Marissa's Story*
## I Am an Oral Person

---

Marissa is a self-proclaimed chatterbox. "I'm always talking," she told me. Marissa explained that she always felt she needed to keep her mouth moving, and she realized she often kept it moving not only by talking, or by chewing on the top of pens (a habit since middle school), but by eating. Marissa also said she felt secure by carrying around a water bottle all day. She got a sense of comfort not so much from the hydration, but more from the ability to be able to take a swig at any time. Marissa learned to accept the fact that she was an oral person. She needed to take that quality and turn it into weight-loss support, instead of sabotage. We set up an eating plan that worked for Marissa, with plenty of fiber-rich fruits and vegetables to provide a lot of chewing, which she also found to be a stress reliever. With three meals and two snacks planned for each day, Marissa was secure in the fact that she had a stable eating plan.

We also developed a workable exercise regimen, with a forty-five-minute brisk walk daily, so her BEAM Box was filling up. To satisfy her oral urges, Marissa added some mini-tools to keep her mouth busy with very few calories. She bought a variety of sugar-free mints and gum, and relied on those for times she just wanted to have something in her mouth. A favorite flavor was cinnamon, because it provided a jolt to her taste buds. She hardly chewed the gum after it was in her mouth, but rather had it tucked in the side of her jaw. She knew it was there, and it kept her satisfied. She also continued to carry around her bottle of water and added seltzer to her list of favorites, as she enjoyed the fizz for a change. Her between-meal grazing dropped dramatically, as Marissa said she knew her eating had not been because she was hungry. By admitting to herself that she was an oral person, Marissa had found some small but effective tools for herself. When it comes to building a toolbox, no tool or crutch is too small. If it helps you, it's a winner.

---

## Boredom

Eating food has become an activity, replacing others that require more thought. The boredom eater is never hungry, since food is consumed regularly throughout the day and night. Finding activities to replace eating (and use your hands) is the key to managing here.

If you eat to stop your boredom, here are four constructive ways to handle this impulse:

- Learn to knit or crochet.
- Clean out a drawer.

- Telephone a friend.
- Brush your teeth.

### Jane's Story
## I'm Bored, So I Eat

Jane was refreshingly honest when she described her weight problems. "My children are now both in college, and I don't really have enough to do. I'm sixty years old, and I've gained eighteen pounds in the past year, and it's getting worse." She did daily volunteer work with her church and thought she was busy enough, but felt stuck and in a rut. When we reviewed Jane's food log, it became clear that her boredom eating occurred mainly in the late afternoon. That was her down time between her morning volunteerism and preparing dinner for her husband, who returned home from his job as an accountant around six o'clock. She was grazing for about three hours a day, between the hours of two and five. She alternated between watching talk shows, talking on the phone, and reading magazines, all the while mindlessly grazing in her cabinets and fridge.

For Jane, we added both structure and a change of scenery to change this pattern. First, she agreed to go home after her volunteer work around one o'clock and eat lunch. Not interested in cooking at midday, Jane ate a microwavable calorie-controlled lunch followed by a piece of fresh fruit. After lunch she brushed her teeth to signal the completion of her eating episode. She then left the house to run errands, returning after two-thirty. Whether it was buying groceries, window shopping, or browsing in a bookstore, Jane made a point of leaving the house in the afternoon, to create an activity. She also learned a new skill that kept her busy without food: she took up knitting. Jane joined a local knitting group in the evening, where she was surprised to find women and men of all ages attending for different reasons. While Jane isn't tackling any major projects soon, she is happily making scarves and hats for friends and loved ones. She keeps her knitting supplies in the kitchen, by the fridge, and now reaches for her needles instead of a snack. With just these simple changes, based on her own honesty, Jane has lost 12 pounds in the past three months.

---

## Socializing

Like the food lover, the social eater tends to disconnect from monitored eating when around friends and abundant food and drink. It's a chance to indulge so, why not? It's so much fun to do, says the social eater. This problem is easier to manage than the others, since the issue that usually plagues the social eater is volume, not frequency.

If you are a social eater, here are four constructive ways to handle this impulse:

- Replace an alcoholic beverage with seltzer and a squeeze of lime.
- Order two small plates (appetizers) instead of an entrée in a restaurant.
- Be a taster and seek variety in tablespoon-sized portions at buffets.
- Enjoy alcohol? Keep it simple and avoid fruit juice and soda mixers.

### Jack's Story
## When I'm with Friends, I Get Off Track

Twenty-nine years old and single, Jack is a social eater. When he's in a structured routine of home and office during the workweek, he generally stays on track with moderate eating, but he veers off course when socializing with his friends. He first came to me after gradually packing on almost 20 pounds over the course of the last year. He had no health problems at the moment and was optimistic about his weight-loss abilities. In fact, he pointed out that if he did not monitor his eating so closely during the workweek, he'd likely have gained much more than he did. Jack's problem was that whenever he joined his friends to socialize, he just disconnected from his typical habits and overindulged in both food and alcohol. As an architect, Jack is fairly sedentary during the day, although he does use the gym in his apartment building "on occasion."

Jack wasn't interested in cutting back on his socializing as a way to limit his indulgences; he preferred instead to moderate what he did, several times a week, to rein in his calories, lose some weight, and keep it from creeping up again. Jack divided his week into weekdays (work time) and weekends (leisure time). If he went out during the week (Monday through Thursday) with friends, he would limit himself to one alcoholic beverage (he chose a martini) and avoid the bar food prior to the meal. He asked for extra olives in his drink, to serve as a mini-appetizer. If the group extended their cocktail hour, he ordered club soda and lime for his second drink. For his meal he ordered two small plates, rather than a large entrée. This worked for Jack, because he agreed that no one was watching what he ate or drank, and his socializing was just as enjoyable regardless of what or how much he ate. It was up to *him* to make better choices, and not expect the group to change.

Jack wanted to loosen up on his weekend socializing, but he also agreed to exercise more. He went on the treadmill for an hour on Saturdays and Sundays, to barter for extra weekend calories. He was satisfied to continue his workweek eating limits, but preferred to allow himself additional alcoholic beverage calories. Since he had cut back to one cocktail during the week, allowing himself two cocktails on weekend evenings felt like a significant indulgence. Another inclusion to his weekend eating strategy was to order grilled fish and vegetables instead of two small plates and to indulge in a dessert by sharing one with three other people.

Because these were all modest changes, Jack understood that he needed to be consistent in order to lose weight. As a social eater, Jack took this new plan seriously and he dropped 10 pounds in about three months. His success has given him confidence, and right now, he's happy to go along at his modest rate of weight loss, which he can sustain with moderate, but not heroic, effort. He does not feel deprived of food or of social activity. A win-win for Jack over the long term.

## Lack of Control

People who lack control over their eating most often say, *"I'm* out of control." Because their entire life feels out of control, it's not just eating that has to be addressed, it's all of the other factors contributing to the out-of-control eater's sense of helplessness over the situation.

If you eat because you feel your life is out of control, here are four constructive ways to respond to this impulse.

- Simplify your life and learn to say no to others.
- Set aside thirty minutes every day just for you. Walk, read the paper, watch the news, window shop, or just sit and relax in blissful silence.
- Create structure in your day, including a plan to eat regularly, three or four times a day.
- Ask for help. You may need friends, family, or professionals to help you retool your daily life.

### *Diane's Story*
## My Life Is Out of Control

As an attorney, mom, wife, daughter, sister, and volunteer—"Not necessarily in that order," she adds—Diane is pulled in fifty different directions on a good day. She is always eating on the run, skipping meals during the day and eating late at night when she feels more relaxed. She felt she could not control her eating. When we met, Diane's weight had been steadily climbing for the past decade, and she had put 30 pounds onto her five-foot-three-inch frame. Her clothes didn't fit, and though she was in good health, she felt defeated by her inability to get control of her eating.

Diane and I had an open and honest discussion about what exactly was out of control. It really wasn't her eating, but rather her present lifestyle. Diane knew what to do—how to eat for weight loss, how to balance—but things were now beyond her tipping point, and she needed help. She agreed that she needed to get her life back under *her* control, rather than always feeling that she was struggling to keep up. A generally happy and optimistic woman, Diane, at forty-three, didn't like this feeling, and feared she was going down an unhealthy road to continuing weight gain and health problems.

Diane made a list of the ways she could delegate her present tasks. First, she learned to say no to a variety of requests, ranging from school volunteerism to selected household activities. Her response became, "Sorry, not this time," to leave the option open to say yes some other time in the future. She would purchase cookies from a bakery for school bake sales, instead of baking at ten o'clock at night, her first free moment of the day. She turned to meal replacements for breakfast (a bar) and for lunch (a shake), and added a fruit with each, to provide structured eating during her busy workday. She carved out thirty minutes in the late afternoon just for herself. It was up to her whether she would use it for a power walk, a stroll in the bookstore, a phone call with a friend, putting her feet up with a cup of herbal tea, or some other activity that was pleasurable for her. She agreed it was not a waste of time, but was important to recharge her personal batteries.

While she and her husband both worked full-time outside of the home, Diane had been reluctant to ask her husband to help with household activities; now she worked out a plan with him to help her whenever she needed it. She wasn't comfortable with a fixed set of chores for him, but she made the big mental leap of asking him for help. Diane was surprised at how soon she felt better, and she regained a sense of control. It was reflected, she said, in not having a "pit in my stomach" most of the time. Feeling less burdened, she was able to focus more on her own reasons for eating and her physical activity. She found that her thirty personal minutes were the best time for a walk. During the first month of her plan, Diane lost only 2 pounds, but she gained a lot of confidence. By the end of seven months, she'd lost a total of 25 pounds. While Diane had a strong set of lifestyle tools and did know what to do to lose weight, she needed to first regain control of her day, to make her BEAM Box effective.

## 4. Turn Good Intentions into Successful Change

We all have many good intentions, but we often sabotage ourselves when it comes to goal setting. The bar is set way too high with expectations for lifestyle changes that are just not sustainable for the long term and wind up lasting only a week or two. You've got to add the tool of *effective* goal setting, which takes a little more thought. I like to separate goals into "perfect world" (unrealistic) goals and "real world" (realistic) goals. We all make fantastic promises to ourselves, but when real life intervenes and derails our good intentions, it can seriously demoralize us. Your strategy should be to set goals that will work in the real world, not the perfect one. Once you've agreed to that plan, your tools will fall right into place. Here are many of my favorites. Once you get started, you'll be able to think of many others that work for you.

### The Perfect World versus the Real World

*Perfect world*: Never eat after 7 p.m.
*Real world*: Allow one mini-meal at night (up to 200 calories).

*Perfect world*: Avoid all fast food.
*Real world*: Choose a kid's meal.

*Perfect world*: Visit the gym every day.
*Real world*: Go to the gym at least three days a week.

*Perfect world*: Cook a low-calorie dinner every night.
*Real world*: Keep calorie-controlled frozen entrées on hand.

*Perfect world*: Eliminate a late-afternoon snack to save calories.
*Real world*: Plan your dinner hour and allow yourself 100 to 200 calories when dinner is two or three hours away.

*Perfect world*: Walk and/or jog four miles on the treadmill daily.
*Real world*: Wear a pedometer and monitor your steps during your daily living activity. Make up the daily difference on the treadmill (10,000 steps is about four miles).

Once you've mastered the best tools for personal goal setting, you'll be able to incorporate your own good intentions into the Real You plan.

## 5. Make One Change at a Time to Keep Your Confidence Up

It's so easy to fall into the rut of an all-or-nothing approach to change. I call it the "negative cycle" of change. Making too many changes at once becomes overwhelming; it's too much work, and we just quit. Sound familiar? You want to change this to a positive cycle of change. Identify one change you want to make—not necessarily the one others say is most health promoting!—and do it for one week. Here's a list of small basic changes you'll want to try. I call them "mini-tools." Select one, and make that change every day—consistency is important. After one week, incorporate another one.

## Mini Eating Tools

- Read food labels.
- Write down what you eat.
- Eat five fruits or vegetables each day.
- Have a meatless meal two times during the week.
- Take a daily multiple vitamin/mineral supplement (100% RDI).
- Use reduced-fat dairy products.
- Choose fiber-rich starches.
- Eat fish (fresh or frozen) once a week.
- Have fresh fruit for dessert.
- Buy single-serve ice cream treats under 150 calories per serving.
- Leave a little food on your plate after each meal.

## Mini Physical Activity Tools

- Wear a pedometer and monitor your daily steps.
- Aim for a total of thirty minutes of movement daily (even if only five minutes at a time).
- Stand instead of sit when cooking, reading, talking.
- Walk instead of stand—on the telephone, talking with a coworker.
- Carry your own groceries.
- Hide the TV remote control.
- Wash your car yourself.
- Be inefficient—make multiple trips on your home stairs.
- Take more stairs—even one flight can help.
- Put on some music and dance while you cook or clean.

You get the idea. One change that you can stick with is empowering, and it convinces the most important person of all—you—that you can make a change. When you make small changes over time, and not big ones all at once, you've created manageable and sustainable expectations for yourself. As with so many other things in life, with weight loss, slow and steady wins the race.

## 6. Use Food to Help Manage Emotional Stress

Food can and should be a tool to help relieve emotional stress. What? How can I say that in a weight-loss book? Isn't the goal to conquer stress eating? I think it is possible to manage stress eating and to be prepared for when it strikes. We all know that food is soothing, and that's the problem with stress eating. Going overboard and losing control are where the problem lies. It's a matter of choosing a small amount of the right kind of food that will control and soothe, without triggering overeating. This concept takes some thought. The mental battle of not eating is often won by consuming about 100 to 200 calories of a preferred (treat) food— but not one that is a trigger. Choose a food that will satisfy, but is not too tasty to resist overeating.

### *Terry's Story*
### I Like to Eat in the Evening

Terry's story was a familiar one to me—it involves one of the "old wives' tales" of weight loss. "I can manage during the day, but I really enjoy eating in the evening and can't seem to control it." She went on to say that she knew it was bad to eat after dinner, and that this was probably the sole cause of her weight struggles. While unmonitored evening eating is often a major cause of excessive calorie consumption, eating after dinner can be included, if you preplan. Terry was already doing a lot of things right. She was a structured eater and paced her breakfast, lunch, and dinner. She included a midmorning and a late-afternoon snack. She ate dinner between six-thirty and seven and went to bed around midnight. That's where, as she put it, "I got into trouble." Since Terry thought it was wrong to eat after dinner, she tailored her eating to what she felt she was supposed to be doing, rather than what was realistic for her. She agreed that she enjoyed evening eating, as it was a relaxing part of the day for her, and she looked forward to it. Right now, though, she could not reconcile this evening eating with effective weight loss.

We reviewed Terry's overall eating plan and made two changes to address her evening eating: First, she agreed to adjust her eating pattern to make her dinnertime a little later; and second, she allowed herself 200 "free calories" of her choice each evening. To make this work, Terry did some bartering. She eliminated her 100-calorie midmorning snack, which she had been eating because she felt she should refuel between breakfast and lunch, even though she was not hungry. She maintained the same lunch, and she was content with it even without having eaten the midmorning snack. She also pushed back her afternoon snack (usually a low-fat cheese stick and a 100-calorie whole grain cracker pack) by an hour, to four o'clock. This allowed her to then hold off on eating dinner until seven-thirty or eight, after which she could still indulge with her new evening calorie allowance. So her caloric bartering provided for some extra calorie consumption at the time she needed it.

All Terry needed to do was preplan and adjust her eating for a modest calorie indulgence in the evening, when she really enjoyed the calories. Her guilt about evening eating was gone, and Terry was now confident that she could finally control it. She was right. Allowing herself a modest caloric load (200 calories) saved her about 500 calories a day from her evening "grazing." That became a weight loss of 1 pound a week. She turned weight creep into steady weight loss with a realistic, practical, and guilt-free approach

---

## 7. Recognize Trigger Foods and Agree to Avoid Them

When it comes to trigger foods, everyone has their own. There is never any hesitation when I'm asked that question. For me, it's pistachio nuts. The difference between a trigger food and one that you simply like a lot is that, with a trigger food, it's too tough to eat just a little. As most people describe it, "Once I start eating, I can't stop." If it's so easy to identify your trigger foods, why is it so hard to avoid them? Because we don't establish substitutes for these foods, as a compromise. We think of these foods as all or nothing. Step one is easy: recognize your trigger foods. Step two is the challenge: find substitutes that provide the same emotional support, with fewer calories and less temptation to overeat them.

Forget about whether that temptation is due to behavior (yes!) or biology (no!), and just learn to manage it. Remember that you're not a better person because you can conquer your food triggers. Sometimes you just need to avoid your potential triggers. You can revisit these foods periodically, to see if you've developed better strategies for control. All you need is to have one alternative to satisfy, and to know which other options need to be avoided. Using myself as an example, with pistachio nuts being my personal trigger, I've found that buying the single-serve 120-calorie pack of pistachios *in their shells* works for me. I only found this solution recently, after months (years?) of struggling, when the individual packs became available. I can visualize the whole portion in its lovely package, and I can eat the whole thing. On the other hand, I do recognize that I must avoid pistachios in bulk baskets—I feel like diving head-first into the giant displays sometimes found in supermarkets—large bags, or the worst for me, already shelled, ready-to-eat kernels.

When it comes to trigger foods, the goal is to satisfy without triggering overeating. Calorie-wise, about 100 to 150 calories provide biological as well as mental satisfaction. It's important to avoid deprivation, because the more you say no to a particular food, the more deprived you feel, and then you become more likely to lose control and overeat. By managing your trigger foods, you'll gain confidence by being in control and feeling satisfied. Achieving that control takes a little personal experimentation. One person's guaranteed solution is someone else's major trigger!

Here are four major groups of trigger foods, and some of my favorite substitutions that might work for you. You'll notice that the list includes both "fun foods" and healthful choices. Think of it as a starter list, to which you add your own favorites. What's most important here is contentment and satisfaction, with caloric control. Give it a try.

**Trigger: Chocolate**

25-calorie, sugar-free hot chocolate mix (Nestlé or Swiss Miss)

3 chocolate-covered strawberries

60-calorie Jell-O sugar-free chocolate pudding

4 Hershey Kisses, dark or milk chocolate

100-calorie bag of M&M's, or chocolate sticks (all brands)

Any 90- to 100-calorie "fun size" candy bar

Mini-bar of Lindt 70 percent dark chocolate

2 mini Tootsie Rolls

100-calorie pack of Nabisco Oreo crisps

100-calorie pack of Hostess mini chocolate cupcakes

Single-stick Fudgesicle (regular, not sugar-free or fat-free)

3 pieces chocolate licorice

2 Altoid chocolate-covered mints

100-calorie bag Emerald Cocoa Roast almonds

**Trigger: Anything with a sweet taste**

Any fresh, ripe fruit (nature's candy)

1 cup of frozen cherries (right from the freezer)

100-calorie bag of Craisins or raisins

Stretch Island fruit leather

Freeze-dried fruits

Single-serve bag of dried apricots or plums

Individually wrapped Sunkist prune

1 Dum Dum lollipop

1 individually wrapped Life Saver

1 Tootsie Pop

100-calorie pack of Swedish fish candy, fruit chews, or strips

Single-wrapped Twizzler

Mini-box of Hot Tamales candy

Dentyne Fire Cinnamon sugar-free gum (or other sugar-free cinnamon gum)

Dried ginger chips

### Trigger: Anything with a salty taste or crunchy texture

Large, crisp dill pickle

Fresh celery with fat-free ranch dip

Single-serve bag (100 calories) of Popchips

100-calorie microwavable popcorn, plain, butter, or kettle flavored

Smartfood single-serve White Cheddar Cheese popcorn

100 calorie bag Cape Cod reduced-fat potato chips

Single-serve bag of Baked Lay's potato chips

15 Triscuit Thin Crisps or Reduced Fat Wheat Thins

1 salted hard Dutch pretzel (caution: strong teeth needed!)

### Trigger: Anything smooth and creamy (that is, with fat)

Nonfat Greek-style yogurt (any brand)

Single serve nonfat, sugar-free yogurt (any flavor)

Kozy Shack sugar-free rice pudding

60-calorie Jell-O sugar-free vanilla (or other flavored) pudding

Weight Watchers Giant Latte ice cream bar and other novelty frozen products (150 calories or less)

Skinny Cow novelty frozen products

Small 2% milk latte

Small (½ cup) Dairy Queen or Tasti D-lite soft-serve dish

Single serve Edy's low-fat ice cream (any flavor)

Small (½ cup) low-fat vanilla or green tea frozen yogurt (no toppings)

## 8. Reward Yourself without Using Food

Another effective tool is finding other ways to reward yourself without using food. As with all of these behavioral tools, the choice is unique to you. One person's perfect treat is some else's toxic nightmare. While it might be a private yoga session or a new bike, it might also be a new lipstick, an expensive haircut, or a spa treatment. The most important insight here is to replace food as the reward with something you can't eat, but can still enjoy. You might also indulge in an expensive, low-calorie edible as a reward—the perfect locally grown berries, or exotic baby lettuce, or an unusual imported red wine vinegar. We have been taught for so long that food is a reward, and it can serve that role at times. But if weight loss is your goal, you'll have to frequently add non-food rewards to the mix.

## 9. Address Your Life-Coping Skills

Addressing your life-coping skills is one of the toughest tools to incorporate in your BEAM Box. It's very hard to accept that food might be your chosen method of coping with life and its daily problems. Without a doubt, life is a lot more complicated and tough than it was twenty years ago, or even five to ten years ago. No wonder the rate of obesity is climbing astronomically. If you find that you're turning to food to avoid your problems, it's time to think about getting some professional help. While many people have a trusted friend or relative to help with emotional support, others feel alone, even when surrounded by people. I'm not only talking about having a weight loss buddy, but suggesting that you find a support group, therapy group, or private counselor to help you get some insights into how to better manage your daily life. With that extra support, you'll be able to better limit your dependence on food and structure a healthier relationship with eating.

Needing extra support doesn't mean you're weak or have no willpower, it only means that life is complex. Having some help in managing life's problems is often directly connected with your ability to moderate your eating in response to real-life stressors. Selecting this tool is an indication of strength, not weakness—as many mistakenly think—and shows a willingness to have some help in building the most effective behavioral tools to long-term weight loss.

## 10. Weigh Yourself Regularly

It's important to view the scale not as the enemy, but as just one tool to help monitor your progress. While some folks have thrown away their scales and don't worry about the pounds—you may know some of them!—it's not a strategy that works for most people. Research studies show clearly that regular weighing is important to long-term weight loss and maintenance.

Getting on the scale daily or weekly helps keep you on track. Regular weighing also allows you to see a number for what it is—an index of your current progress. It's one of the most important tools to fight weight creep, the pounds that slowly sneak up over time.

# Fernstrom Fundamentals

Now that you're warmed up with the first ten tools, I've got a dozen more for you! Let's turn for a minute to some other areas of self-awareness and an even more thorough framework for goal-setting.

I've distilled most of the behavioral tools into an easy set of fundamentals upon which you can establish a strong basis for success. These twelve tools are a must-have for all toolboxes, to help you prepare for any challenging situation. These tools will become a workhorse to be pulled out frequently, often in combination.

You'll have a three-pronged behavioral approach that will allow you to:

- Conquer your old barriers preventing weight loss success.
- Maintain motivation and focus.
- Develop lifestyle moderation. (Avoid extreme behaviors.)

1. **Stay connected.** The Real You plan is a lifestyle, not a diet. It may not seem different at first, but you can go "on" and "off" a

FERNSTROM FUNDAMENTALS

*Twelve Behavioral Tools for Long-Term Weight-Loss Success*

1. Stay connected.
2. Think before you eat anything.
3. Recognize contentment: Aim for "Level 2" of fullness.
4. Minimize mindless eating.
5. Agree that there are no bad foods, just bad portions.
6. Learn to barter.
7. Keep your mouth busy with non-calorie activities.
8. Buy single servings.
9. Accept your temperament.
10. Remind yourself that daily physical activity is important.
11. Wear a pedometer.
12. Don't beat yourself up; Learn from your mistakes.

diet. You are in a lifestyle for *life*. When you choose to stay connected, it only means that you choose not to disconnect from your plan totally. We have all faced times when we just want to blow it all off and worry about things next week, next month, or next year. When you stay connected, it means that you will focus on avoiding a sabotage of uncontrolled eating, and minimize the caloric damage. One health-promoting activity a day, minimum, will ensure that you are connected—whether it's eating five fruits and veggies or a taking a twenty-minute walk. Always know that on some days you are more connected than on others. It's like flying a kite: sometimes it's way up in the clouds and you can't see it, but it's still just as connected as when it's just above you.

2. **Think before you eat anything.** The best way to stay connected is to think before you eat. This doesn't mean don't eat. It means

make a better choice. So often we don't stop to think, and then we overeat, only later wondering why we did it. If you choose to think before you eat, you can buy yourself some time to make a better choice. It might be grilled chicken instead of a burger, or it might be one cookie instead of two. If you think before you eat, you will *always* make a better choice.

3. **Recognize contentment. Look for Level 2 of fullness.** We all eat to what I call "Level 3" of fullness in our culture—until we are stuffed. How many times have we eaten until we feel like we're going to burst? Level 3 means we are physically unable to eat any more. So, how to recognize Level 2—meaning you are content and satisfied, but you *could eat more?* That's the new end point that you must accept in order to lose weight and keep it off. Here's the challenge: *choosing to listen to that signal.* The flip side of this, to avoid feeling deprived, is to tell yourself, "There's always more food later." The question we all fear when we stop at contentment—that uneasy feeling at first—is, "What if I'm hungry later?" The answer: "I'll eat later." You will find that, surprisingly, a more modest number of calories will return you to Level 2 of fullness. It will take 100 to 200 calories to satisfy, rather than 900 to 1,000.

4. **Minimize mindless eating.** So often we eat without thinking—what I call "mindless eating." It is so easy to do, and it does take effort to learn how to manage it. If you are aware that you do this, make a mental note and gradually change the behavior. First, always think before anything goes into your mouth. Decide whether you are hungry, thirsty, or simply bored. You can take a step back and decide to have a low-calorie beverage or snack, or pursue a nonfood activity (like cleaning a drawer or knitting).

5. **Agree that there are no bad foods, just bad portions.** This is a fundamental you must embrace for long-term success. It's hard in this culture of "good" versus "bad" foods, with all of its definitions and explanations of what makes something good or bad. Baloney. The old phrase "everything in moderation" is most true when it comes to food. There is no food that is off-limits forever. That knowledge is the key to maintaining control, and reducing

the pressure of food restriction is necessary for long-term weight control. A taste is as good as a large serving. When you learn to be a taster, you can make food work for you more effectively. The first bite or two is always the most satisfying—and when you limit your consumption to a small serving, you will enjoy it fully.

While there are certainly no bad foods, there may be selected items that you personally find difficult to limit. For those items, it's likely best to eliminate them for a short period of time—out of sight, out of mind—and retry now and then, if you feel you'd like to include them. Rather than eliminate those foods, substitute other foods over which you have better control. For example, if you love nuts but find it hard to limit your serving size, substitute a single-serving bag of light microwave popcorn. Let your imagination be your guide.

6. **Learn to barter.** Bartering is one of the best tools you have to avoid deprivation. Whether you do this on a daily or weekly basis, you can take the pressure off by *choosing* one food over another— you have control over the food. "I will choose a roll and skip the potato," or "I will have a glass of wine and skip the dessert," or "I will share a dessert and skip the roll"—you get the idea. When you provide the choice for yourself, it becomes easier to see that there is no deprivation in your lifestyle, only prioritizing what you eat at a particular time. You can always make a different choice later on.

7. **Keep your mouth busy with noncalorie items.** There may not be a free lunch, but there are some "freebies" you can pull out of your toolbox to help you stay on track. The best ammunition for "head hunger" are things like water, seltzer, low-calorie drinks, and sugarless mints and sugarless gum, all of which keep your mouth busy with almost no calories (see the Anytime Foods and Drinks in chapter 7). Sometimes it's not enough to "just say no" to food, and the helpful tool of keeping your mouth busy with a noncalorie item can help get you through a difficult time. We all have them.

8. **Buy single servings.** Single servings cost more, but they provide automatic portion control and way more satisfaction—that sense of

eating to the bottom of the bag. Whether it's a mini-bag of popcorn, a mini candy bar, a small, prewrapped piece of low-fat cheese, or a prepackaged meal, it really takes the pressure off to know that you can eat the whole thing. It is also a major help in learning when the meal or snack is done. You can preplan and determine that your single serving is all that you will consume, and when it is done, there is no more. Even if you do not feel content, limiting yourself to a single serving can help with portion control.

9. **Accept your temperament.** You are who you are. Sounds silly, but when you take a step back and analyze yourself, it's easy to see the highs and lows of your eating personality. Identify when you are most vulnerable—late afternoon and evening are common times—and minimize the caloric damage you may do at that time. If you are someone (like me) who is an evening eater and really enjoys food a couple of hours after dinner, then preplan for these times with modest calories. This approach is another type of bartering: saving some calories for your vulnerable times to relieve the pressure. In order to be successful here, you will need to take a good look at your lifestyle patterns to recognize when you're struggling and when you're managing well.

10. **Remind yourself that daily physical activity is important.** So often we focus only on the caloric intake part of the weight-loss equation. Daily physical activity is not only important, it is essential to long-term weight management. We have many barriers to physical activity—and I don't mean running a marathon. I mean making the habit of regular daily activity. Some days may be more active than others, but having the mind-set to keep moving is critical. If you learn to make this a priority, no matter what your level ability, you will make time to increase what I call your "activity of daily living." We can all park farther away from the market, take one flight of stairs, walk up the escalator, take the dog for a walk. Physical activity doesn't always mean an aerobics class or an hour on the treadmill. Even five minutes six or seven times a day is a health promoter.

11. **Wear a pedometer.** We often cannot separate mental fatigue from physical fatigue. We can have a very stressful day and think

we feel physically exhausted. The best way to determine your daily activity is to wear a pedometer and count your steps. Remember that it takes about 2,500 steps to make a mile, which is also about 100 calories. Keep that in mind when you think about activity. An extra 5,000 steps added to your day (about forty minutes of walking) can save 200 calories. That's a big help on the energy balance end. Exercise alone, without reducing intake, rarely results in significant weight loss, but combined with modest food restriction, it is the key tool to sustained weight loss and maintenance.

12. **Don't beat yourself up; learn from your mistakes.** Losing weight is very tough. If it were easy, everyone would be thin. When it comes to losing weight, we are highly critical of ourselves. You need to think of this as your own weight-loss journey. Sometimes it's easy to lose focus, but that does not mean you have failed. It means you need to take a step back and evaluate why you feel things are not going as you expected. When your expectations do not meet your goals, whether it's rate of weight loss, or restaurant choices, or selections at a family barbecue, do not get down on yourself. Life is not perfect, and neither are we. Move on, and try to see what made you more vulnerable at the time of the lapse. It might not be perfect the next time it occurs (and it will happen again), but you will be better able to recognize the vulnerability, and maintain better control. You do not need to be perfect, only to make your best effort at control. And when you lose it (which happens sometimes), you regroup, and move forward. No looking back.

# Two Final Tools

## Rate Your Effort Level and Avoid Burnout

How hard should it be to make these changes? How much effort is enough? We always feel we should be working harder at weight loss, no matter what our effort—and that's not realistic. Use this easy ten-point

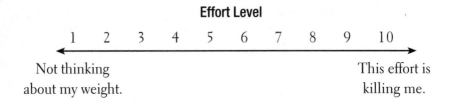

**Effort Level**

1    2    3    4    5    6    7    8    9    10

Not thinking                                            This effort is
about my weight.                                        killing me.

scale to help you figure out your optimal long-term effort for weight loss. On a scale from 1 to 10, where 1 is "I'm not working at weight loss at all," and 10 is "Ugh, this is so hard, I can't keep this up for longer than a week," mark off where you are on most days. Your effort level needs to be around 5 or 6 daily, for consistent weight loss. Only you can gauge what your maximal effort is. Everyone's is different. If you're losing weight at a rapid clip, and rating a 10, then this is only going to be a temporary strategy for you, and you must modify your rate of weight loss for the long term. Heroic effort is not sustainable for the long term.

This rating also comes in handy when it comes to picking a target weight. If your effort level is at 5 or 6 every day, and you're at a weight that is sustainable, then learn to be happy there. If maintaining your weight takes a 9 or 10 effort level daily, you're likely to set yourself up for disappointment in time. Sometimes it's only a matter of 2 or 3 pounds to take your effort level from a 9 to a 6! You have to ask yourself what the *personal cost* is to you, to keep up an effort that is just too difficult to maintain a weight. Learn to live in a size 10 body (level 6 effort) and not a size 6 (level 10 effort). It's okay to be a man with a 36-inch waist (level 5.5 effort) instead of a 34 incher (level 9 effort). It's all about effort level. That's a difficult mental leap, but one that is manageable, once you see where you fall on the "effort-level" line.

## Avoid Boredom: When to Switch Tools

Often we hit a wall when we've been doing well with a lifestyle plan but it has become tedious, boring, and hard to maintain. Most people panic at that point, thinking something must be wrong. I disagree. I think it's the perfect opportunity for you to reevaluate what you've been doing and reward yourself for the good behaviors you've sustained by taking a break and shaking up your plan a little bit. I don't mean stop your positive behaviors that serve you well. I mean it's time to introduce some new tools, as temporary replacements or alternatives to prevent boredom and keep your plan fresh. Whether it's swapping a high-protein breakfast for a fiber-rich starch replacement, or taking a break from your home treadmill to walking the mall or department store, it's up to you to *recognize* when boredom is setting in. Structure and repetition are great parts of your toolbox, but there's a fine line between repetition and boredom. Boredom might sneak up on you once a month, or once a year; but once you recognize it's happening, you won't get stuck!

### *Barbara's Story*
## I'm Sick of My Plan

When she came to see me, Barbara sounded like someone with the perfect plan. She knew what worked for her, and she could stick with it. She'd lost 15 pounds, and for health reasons (she had high blood pressure) she needed to lose another 10 pounds. She felt good about her efforts, but in the past few weeks it had become harder for her to stay on track. She found reasons why she couldn't get to the gym, where she'd been a regular on the elliptical machines three times a week for forty minutes. She felt that she was slipping in her eating plan, and it took a huge amount of personal effort to not cheat. Barbara acknowledged that she really was just sick of her plan—which had worked so well for her—and she was questioning her ability to stay on track on her own. That's when she came to see me.

Barbara had had success with a high-protein plan that also focused on heart-healthy fats. While she did consume some carbohydrates, mostly vegetables and limited fruits, she typically avoided all starchy carbohydrates. She had been on her plan for months, and now found she couldn't stand the thought of eating protein, such as eggs or cottage cheese, for breakfast, and even dreamed of waffles with syrup or a large muffin. We agreed her dreams were telling her something. As humans who used to forage for food, before we only had to go as far as the local supermarket, it is part of our biology to seek variety in the foods we eat.

We are hard-wired to choose a variety of foods, to ensure we meet all of our nutritional requirements. The solution for Barbara was an easy one, once she overcame her fear that she would gain weight by adding any starchy carbohydrates. She agreed that calories were what counted, and that if she chose a limited number of starchy carbohydrates, rich in protein and fiber, she would find her effort level returning to an acceptable, not heroic, level. She simply needed a little variety. Barbara replaced her routine breakfast of an egg-white omelet with a single-serve packet of Weight Control instant oatmeal with some added berries. At lunch, she added a thin wrap (about 100 calories) to her daily salad of mixed greens and sliced chicken.

For her evening snack, instead of a yogurt, she ate a 100-calorie bag of microwave popcorn. This simple option provided enough variety for Barbara when she felt she needed a change. She did not have to eat these starchier items with mandatory frequency, and she listened to her body. She had variety, with control. Her effort level returned to one that was manageable, and she was also surprised to find that her interest in the gym and the elliptical machine returned. In fact, Barbara was now also prepared to shake up her gym routine and attend a class if she started losing interest again. The addition to Barbara's BEAM Box was a little variety. Her plan had become rigid, resulting in an effort level that was not sustainable over time. She lost her last 10 pounds, and has been able to keep the extra weight off for the past two years, all by knowing not only when, but how, to tweak her plan to avoid boredom and burnout.

# 4

# Eating and Food Tools
## Choosing What to Eat

**While the food we eat** is a major tool in everyone's toolbox, we often make the mistake of thinking it's the only one that really counts and that all the other tools are much less important by comparison. To lose weight and keep it off, you've first got to accept that food intake alone is *not* the master tool leading to long-term successful weight loss. Drastic reductions in calories can produce quick, but not permanent, weight loss. For your food tools to be a success, they must work in a partnership with the kind of person you are, the kinds of changes you are both willing and able to make, and your own relationship history with food.

What is the best eating plan for weight loss? I'm asked this question every day. While the foundation is biologically based on reducing the calories ingested daily, my answer is always the same: a plan that keeps you interested, and provides *structure* without *rigidity*. Think about this for a minute.

What's the difference, you might ask? I say there's a big one. *Rigidity* means that you have such a strict eating plan that if you vary a little you'll go off the deep end. Many people are afraid of veering out of control, so they become rigid eaters, thinking (incorrectly) that they have good control. *Structure* means that your plan has a little flexibility—you give yourself a little wiggle room. Only structured eating leads to success and long-term control. If you're a rigid eater, you always worry about getting off track, and your worries put a lot of pressure on you. Even worse, when you get off track, the whole plan collapses and you feel like a failure. Not this time! With the Real You plan, you will tailor your food tools to work *for* you, instead of *against* you!

This chapter explains the seventeen basic tools you can use to become a structured eater and maintain your weight loss over the long term. You'll notice that some of these overlap with the behavior tools described in chapter 3. That's not surprising, since choosing what to eat is not just about hunger and healthy choices but also relates to your attitude and environment.

## 1. Bite and Write: Lifestyle Logging

While it sounds simple, it's hard for most people to keep track of their daily eating. If you feel the need to skip over this section, having done this "dozens of times," go ahead and do it. There's nothing magical about writing down what you eat—you don't automatically eat less. But the one thing that logging does is force you to think before you eat anything. What I like about lifestyle logging is that you're keeping track of not only food intake, but also your activity, your feelings (both positive and negative), and your sleep patterns on a daily basis. I'm a fan of pen and paper logging, because it makes a stronger connection between you and your food intake. For many people, spreadsheets, PDA programs, and online tracking services can work just as well. Whichever tracking method you use, you'll want to make sure your lifestyle log includes these four parts:

Amount and type of food
Duration and intensity of activity

Sleep pattern: quality and amount

Stress management: daily feelings (positive and negative)

You might log for two weeks, two months, or two years. The real goal, for the long term, is to convert this logging to your mental database. Over time, you'll want to use the lifestyle logging now and then as a snapshot of your lifestyle—when you're bored with your plan or feel like you're getting off track.

## 2. Read Food Labels

Nowadays a food label looks like a page from a science textbook—so much information packed into such a small space. While only some of the information is required by law, food factlets turn up everywhere on the box. Is all of this information necessary to read every time you make a choice? In a word, no. That's why I think so many people just give up reading the labels altogether. Others tell me they're actually embarrassed to ask for an easy shortcut to reading food labels. In fact, that's a great idea. The first step is to pay attention to the boxed information on the back of the package, with the specifics of the product. Don't be fooled by large type elsewhere on a package with terms like "a good source of whole grain" or "trans-fat free" or "excellent source of vitamin C." These descriptions are meant to grab your attention—Look at me, I'm a healthy choice!—but it's essential to read below the headlines, and check out the main label. When it comes to losing weight, the two most important bits of information are the *serving size* and the *calories per serving size*.

Next, move on to the total fat content. That's an immediate tip-off of caloric density—that is, how large your serving will be. If you're surprised to see a tiny serving size on the package, then check out the percentage of fat, and you'll likely see a high number (a food with 3 grams or less per serving is considered low-fat). It's up to you to decide whether you want a modest portion of a fat-dense food, or a reduced-calorie version, if available, with a larger portion size. The calories will remain the same, either way.

Another helpful weight-control label fact is fiber content. Since fiber is not digestible, it helps you stay fuller longer, without adding extra calories. Aim for at least 3 grams of fiber per serving (some grains contain up to 8 or 9 grams per serving).

If you're sodium sensitive, pay close attention, and even if you're not, aim for 2,400 milligrams (mg) or less daily. Many prepared foods have close to half your total day's intake in just one serving. Stick with fresh or frozen foods to limit this problem. If you buy products such as canned beans because preparing the dried variety is just too much work, dump them in a strainer and rinse them under running water to cut out a lot of the sodium.

Check out the calcium content, particularly for dairy products and other foods that are calcium-fortified. To know what you're getting, take the milligrams (mg) listed per serving and cut off the zero at the end of the number. So a cup of yogurt with 350 mg of calcium contains 35 percent of your recommended daily intake (about a third). Similarly, a product with 80 mg of calcium per serving—which sounds like a lot, if you're not paying attention—contains a mere 8 percent of your suggested daily intake. The percentage of your daily intake is the number to know.

For fresh foods, or those without a package, buy a comprehensive nutrient composition book, or go online to get the specifics. I have not yet seen a food or product for which I couldn't find complete nutrition information online!

The next big challenge on the food label, even for the most experienced label reader, is understanding labeling terms. Nowadays, manufacturers must adhere to federal guidelines when putting certain labels on packaged foods. Here's an easy reference for you to follow when looking at any kind of prepared food.

When the package says "-free," this means the food contains zero, or almost none, of a specific item *per serving*.

*Fat-free*: less than 1/2 gram of fat per serving

*Calorie-free*: less than 5 calories per serving

*Trans-fat-free*: less than 1/2 gram of trans fat per serving

*Cholesterol-free*: less than 1/2 mg of cholesterol per serving and 2 grams or less of saturated fat per serving

*Sugar-free:* less than ½ gram of sucrose (table sugar) per serving; can contain other sweeteners such as sugar alcohols, which have similar calories to table sugar

*Sodium-free:* less than 5 mg per serving

When the package says "low," this means the food doesn't exceed the nationally approved dietary guidelines *per serving.*

*Low-fat:* 3 grams of fat or less per serving

*Low saturated fat:* 1 gram or less of saturated fat per serving and no more than 15 percent of calories from saturated fat

*Low-cholesterol:* 20 mg or less of cholesterol per serving and 2 grams or less of saturated fat per serving

*Low-calorie:* 40 calories or less per serving

*Low-sodium:* 140 mg or less of sodium per serving

*Very low sodium:* 35 mg or less of sodium per serving

For packaged meats, poultry, and fish:

*Lean:* less than 10 grams of fat, less than 4 grams of saturated fat, *and* less than 95 mg of cholesterol per serving

*Extra-lean:* less than 5 grams of fat, less than 2 grams of saturated fat, *and* less than 95 mg of cholesterol per serving

When the package says "reduced," "less," or "lower," it means the product contains 25 percent less than what is contained in the original version. These terms apply to total fat, saturated fat, cholesterol, calories, sugar, and sodium compared to the regular version.

And finally, "light" or "lite" pertains only to products containing one-third fewer calories *or* 50 percent less fat compared to the original product. But you can't necessarily assume that; you must read the label, because "light" may also be used to describe color or texture, without any change in nutrient content. When used for color or texture, the packaging must clearly state "light in color" to avoid confusion. A funny exception here applies to products that are generally known to the public, including "light brown sugar," which refers only to color and does not need to state that it is a full-calorie product. Yet another reason to be a careful label reader!

## 3. Choose a Realistic Rate of Weight Loss:
## Reverse Calorie Counting

It's important to get a reality check of your projected rate of weight loss. When your goals are modest, you'll never be disappointed. Set your goals based on your life *now*, and avoid comparing to a rate of loss you aimed for five, ten, or even twenty years ago. Choose a pace that's realistic for you at this time in your life.

A great way to start is using what I call "reverse calorie counting." In fact, it's not really counting at all. A mistake many people make is to only eat *up to* a limited number of calories, usually leading to a feeling of deprivation. A better way is to *cut back* on what you're already doing. You still learn the calorie-counting basics, but you lose the pressure of a calorie deadline. Using this strategy:

If you save 100 calories every day, you'll lose about 1 pound a month.

If you save 250 calories a day, you'll lose about 2 pounds a month.

If you save 500 calories a day, you'll lose about 1 pound a week.

If you save 1,000 calories a day, you'll lose about 2 pounds a week.

The tricky part is to start with small changes every day and to keep your lifestyle log. Start with easy changes—without doing an overhaul of your eating plan—by cutting calories out of your present eating. If you take what you're eating every day and trim calories from those meals, you're making a great start to learning how to monitor both your portions and your calories.

If you're really not a reverse calorie counter, you might ask about using a calorie limit. If you feel secure with a daily calorie limit, it's important to use some realistic guidelines. The only way to prevent rigidity in your plan is to accept a daily calorie *range*. For women, use a starting range of 1,400 to 1,600 daily calories. For men, use a starting range of 1,800 to 2,000 calories. Aim for the lower range, but accept the higher range as a successful day. After trying this consistently for a month, adjust by 100 to 200 calories in either direction, depending upon your rate of weight loss *and* your effort level. (See chapter 3 for a discussion of effort level.)

## *Joanne's Story*
## I'm a Walking Calorie Counter

Joanne, one of my patients, was always battling an extra 25 pounds. She had been a lifelong calorie counter until finally she said, "I just can't do that anymore." All her life, Joanne ate up to a specific number of calories. She felt a lot of pressure using that method, and it hadn't worked for her. She felt she was always running out of calories, which made her feel "mentally hungry." Joanne was hesitant at first to try reverse calorie counting, thinking it did not give her the kind of control she was accustomed to with a set limit for calories.

Once Joanne understood the concept and saw how she, herself, could create the structure with better choices for every meal and snack, she was enthusiastic. Using her vast knowledge of calorie contents from years of logging and using an online calorie-counting guide, Joanne trimmed calories from her present eating, to save calories every day. Joanne's greatest surprise was that she did not feel deprived, and she lost about 2 pounds a week for the first two months of her plan, which gave her a 15-pound loss. Joanne learned the way to consistently trim calories without having the pressure of calorie limits. Joanne also agreed that it was a great success to maintain her 15-pound loss, and she reset her final goal. She no longer felt that 25 pounds was her target. She was thrilled with her 15-pound loss and her ability to maintain it with moderate, not heroic effort. Her reverse calorie counting really worked and provided a new-found sense of accomplishment and confidence that she could sustain over the long term.

**Joanne's Old Breakfast (560 calories)**

8-ounce glass OJ (140 calories)

2 packets plain instant oatmeal (320 calories)

Coffee with half and half (100 calories)

SAVINGS: 265 calories

**Trimmed Breakfast (255 calories)**

4-ounce glass OJ with 2 ounces water (70 calories)

1 packet plain instant oatmeal (160 calories)

Coffee with whole milk (25 calories)

| Joanne's Old Lunch (1,100 calories) | Trimmed Lunch (520 calories) |
|---|---|
| Combo meal: | Kid's meal: |
| Whopper or Big Mac (600 calories) | Junior Hamburger (260 calories) |
| Medium French fries (500 calories) | Kiddie French fries (260 calories) |
| Diet soda (0 calories) | Diet soda or water (0 calories) |
| SAVINGS: 580 calories | |

| Joanne's Old Dinner (785 calories) | Trimmed Dinner (585 calories) |
|---|---|
| Tomato soup (60 calories) | Tomato Soup (60 calories) |
| 2 grilled chicken breasts (400 calories) | 1 grilled chicken breast (200 calories) |
| Steamed broccoli (75 calories) | Steamed broccoli (75 calories) |
| Baked potato (100 calories) | Baked potato (100 calories) |
| 5-ounce glass of red wine (150 calories) | 5-ounce glass of red wine (150 calories) |
| SAVINGS: 200 calories | |

TOTAL DAILY SAVINGS: 1,045 calories

## 4. Set Up for Success: Be a Structured Eater

Before you jump into deciding *what* to eat, you want to think about *when* to eat. I don't mean going by the clock; I mean creating structure in your eating day, making sure you have at least three "eating intervals" each day. *Eating intervals? You mean meals?* No, I mean eating intervals. Creating structured eating requires thinking about the intervals between when you eat; it's "anti-clock" eating. You don't want to go too long without eating (more than four hours) or not wait at all between eating episodes (within a hour of the last one). You need to preplan some intervals that are *just right* for you. That's where the lifestyle logging comes in handy yet again. We all have selective memory when it comes to structuring our meals.

## 5. Choose How Often to Eat

There are no metabolic absolutes about how often to eat. You do want to refuel at least every four hours or so, but you *can* eat more often, as long as you're dividing up your daily calorie intake into what I call "eating episodes." There's a big gray area here, and a lot of choice, depending on your own daily habits. With my eating episodes, you can eat anywhere from three times to nine times a day.

Here's how it works. From the biology point of view, you need to eat *a minimum* of three times a day—roughly every four to six hours. Eating three times a day is sufficient to let your body know, metabolically, that the food supply is intact. Remember, we are hardwired from caveman and cavewoman days, when food was not always around. It is important to prevent your body from thinking you're in starvation mode, because that causes it to turn down your metabolism, to protect what your body perceives as preparation for a long period without food. Then, when you do eat, you're over-hungry, since that same metabolic response gives your appetite a super-stimulus, to make sure you eat enough for survival. How often have you skipped a meal (or two), thinking you'll save some calories for later, and when you next eat you feel absolutely ravenous? That's your body's natural mechanism to help you get the nutrients you need to stay alive.

You'll first want to divide your total food consumption into *three* different times of day. The three times will form the foundation of the model. After that, you can spread out your eating over a larger part of the day (more frequent eating) or you can concentrate it in those three times. You can choose from multiple options. Know yourself. For many, it's tiring and tempting to be eating throughout the day. For others, it's the only way to stay on track. This formula also works if you are a night owl and sleep during the day—just reverse the day and night times.

Suppose you prefer to eat three times a day. Your eating episodes might look like this:

*Morning:* 1 cup grapes; 1/2 English muffin with 1 teaspoon peanut butter or almond butter; 1 4-ounce sugar-free yogurt

*Midday:* 1 cup reduced-salt chicken rice soup; 2 slices reduced-calorie whole wheat bread with 3 ounces turkey, lettuce and tomato, mustard; 1 apple

*Evening:* Large green salad with balsamic vinegar, 6 ounces poached salmon, 1 small sweet potato, ½ cup green beans, 8-ounce glass skim milk, 100-calorie pack cookies

If you ate the same foods as above, but with six eating episodes instead of three, you might divide the foods like this:

*Early morning:* Grapes and English muffin with peanut butter

*Midmorning:* 4-ounce yogurt

*Noon:* Chicken rice soup and turkey sandwich

*Midafternoon:* Apple

*Early evening:* Salad, salmon, sweet potato, and green beans

*An hour before bedtime:* Glass of milk and cookies

And if you wanted to spread the same food out over nine eating episodes, you might do it this way:

1. *8:30 a.m.* 1 cup grapes
2. *9:30 a.m.* ½ English muffin with peanut butter
3. *11:30 a.m.* 4-ounce yogurt
4. *1:00 p.m.* Chicken rice soup
5. *2:00 p.m.* Turkey sandwich
6. *3:30 p.m.* Apple
7. *5:30 p.m.* Large green salad
8. *7:00 p.m.* Salmon, sweet potato, green beans
9. *9:00 p.m.* Cookies and milk

## 6. Identify Your Eating Temperament

We all have different ways of thinking about food, which makes us manage our eating differently. Determining your natural inclinations is an important step in defining your own eating plan. When you go with your personal preferences, it's much easier to sustain your changes for the long term. We all make food selections based on the four basic qualities listed below. How do you prioritize these qualities when you eat?

- Nutrient content
- Taste
- Caloric density (calories per ounce)
- Macronutrient composition (mix of carbohydrate, protein, and fat)

## 7. Know Your Eating Style

An eating style is highly personal, and that's where a lot of variations occur among us. Take an honest look at which taste preferences and eating patterns call out to you. Being true to your tendencies will help you identify your personal barriers in managing your food intake. These differences explain why you might struggle when seeing a candy bar, while your friend can easily pass it up. That same friend might be drawn to a pizza parlor five miles away, while you couldn't care less. It's this individual variability that gives you strength—to see that you do have control over a lot of foods and can learn to adapt your eating style to daily life. It's important to understand your eating style, so you can always come up with a Plan B (see next section) when your eating starts out great but gets wobbly during the day. It's all about understanding yourself.

Identify your own eating style. (Check out chapter 3 to learn more on this topic.)

- Do you like sweet tastes?
- Do you prefer the creamy, smooth taste of fatty foods?
- Do you like crunchy foods?
- Do you like salty foods?
- Do you like savory flavors?
- Do you eat anything fat-free, where portion sizes don't count?
- Do you prefer small amounts of real, flavor-intense foods?
- Are you a member of the Clean Plate Club?
- Are you a meal skipper during the day?
- Do you have trouble distinguishing between hunger and fullness?
- Do you keep your mouth busy for oral satisfaction?

## 8. Avoid Portion Distortion: Preplan Your Meals and Snacks

I am a great defender of those who struggle with portion control. Why? In our country, it's hard to determine appropriate serving sizes. With the supersizing of every food in sight, many of us have become "value" minded. How much food can we get for the least money? Value-centered eating is different from budget-minded healthier eating. At restaurants, giant portions of food are served to us practically flopping off the plate. When it comes to fast food, we can supersize for pennies, and combination meals abound. At home, we have giant-size plates—our salad plates are the size of European dinner plates—and we fill them to the brim. It's too difficult mentally to put less food on a plate, because when we do, the portions look skimpy. We *think* that standard portions are not enough food to satisfy us, because we're so used to looking at mega-portions. It's a mind-stomach connection that has to readjust.

When selecting your food, make sure to look for the recommended serving size as a guideline. You can always choose less than the recommended serving. If you keep the mind-set that you can always have more food later—commonly known as seconds—you will struggle less. Smaller portions don't mean deprivation, they only mean smaller portions!

Taking advantage of the wide variety of foods—both healthful and fun—that come in smaller, single-serving packaging is a big plus to relearning portion control—or learning it for the first time! In fact, the main bonus of using meal replacements for many people, as you'll read later on, is that you've got built-in portion control. Plus, save those containers to use as a guide when you're deciding on real-life food portions. (Note: while your local market may have a modest selection of single-serving foods, check Amazon.com for a more complete listing of 100-calorie and other portion-controlled products you can order online by the case.)

While reading labels and using measuring cups and a food scale are all helpful tools to keep you on track, they're often not available when you're away from home. Here are some of my favorite ways to mentally visualize portion sizes of various foods.

## Meats/Nuts/Other Proteins

1 ounce = a DVD
3 ounces = a deck of cards, your computer mouse
4 ounces = a checkbook
1 teaspoon peanut butter = the tip of your thumb
2 tablespoons peanut butter/hummus = a golf ball
1 ounce nuts = a 2-inch-square sticky note

## Fruits/Vegetables

Medium fruit = a tennis ball
1 cup = your balled-up fist
1/2 cup = a tennis ball cut in half
1 cup salad greens = a baseball

## Grains

1 cup cereal or popcorn = a baseball
1 slice bread = a deck of cards
1/2 cup rice = a tennis ball cut in half
1 cup pasta = a light bulb

## Dairy

1 ounce cheese = 3 stacked dice
1/2 ounce cheese = the size of your thumb
1/2 cup ice cream = a tennis ball cut in half
1 cup yogurt = a baseball

## Fats

1 tablespoon of butter, oil, salad dressing = a poker chip

## Snacks

1 ounce = a small handful
1 1/2 ounces = a large handful

Of course, these comparisons help with eyeballing when you can't get a single-serving package. But it's really worth the extra money to look for single servings, since they give you the value-added feeling of eating the whole thing. This is particularly important if you are a member of the Clean Plate Club. And if you do eat a second 100-calorie serving, you're still way ahead of what you'd typically eat if left with a larger portion. My favorite rule of thumb in the 100-calorie department is to limit yourself to one package of a specific item; do not go for seconds of the same food. You'd be amazed at how this really makes you think before deciding on another package (see the Fernstrom Fundamentals in chapter 3).

## Karen's Story
## I'm a Visual Eater

When she first came to see me, Karen, age thirty-eight, knew her major eating sabotage. "If I see it, I eat it." For many years she had been a member of the Clean Plate Club. As she explained, "I never really understood the connection between the food on my plate and the starving people in other parts of the world," a rationale her parents provided as she was growing up. She always felt compelled to finish whatever was on her plate, whether or not she was full. Karen also never felt she could eyeball portions very well, and thought she needed specific visual cues to help reduce her food intake. She had successfully lost the same 30 pounds she currently was struggling with twice over the past six years. Both times, she did it using commercial plans that provided all the food and snacks. Understanding that meal replacements were not the long-term solution for her, Karen wanted to address the portion control issue head on, in adding tools to her BEAM Box. She had tried a food scale in the past and found it cumbersome.

Karen first downsized her plate and silverware. To get started, she bought a set of toddler utensils and a set of toddler dishes (bowls and plates). While another option was to simply use her salad fork, teaspoon, and salad-size plate, Karen preferred to start fresh with these new, separate tools. She also purchased a set of disposable infant spoons for her lunchtime yogurt at work and sometimes ate with chopsticks to further limit her calories per bite. Karen gained confidence by using her past knowledge of portion size and by using utensils that gave her the visual satisfaction of a full plate.

She also was forced to slow down her eating, since the smaller utensils held less food. Karen admitted that the ingrained habit of cleaning her plate was just too tough to change right now and that she was able to downsize more effectively by starting with less food, rather than by leaving food on the plate. That was a great personal insight for her. Plus, she allowed herself several options in a restaurant that were consistent with her plan. While Karen usually ordered two appetizers, or two items from the "small plates" selections (one being a salad), she would also sometimes share an entrée with a dining companion. Or even order an entrée for herself and ask for an extra sharing plate. "I am sharing with myself for later," she laughed, taking the rest home for another meal.

Karen was now confident that she could continue monitoring her eating with her new tools. She lost 20 pounds in five months and even now, she still uses her smaller utensils and plates to ensure continued portion control. While her ultimate goal is to lose another 10 pounds, she is confident in her ability to maintain her 20-pound loss and feels she will not yo-yo again. She's also much less concerned with her rate of loss for those final pounds and even agrees that she is pleased with her weight loss, even if she has not lost any further weight.

---

## 9. Barter and Exchange Food: Mealtime Strategies

As human eaters, we seek variety, which is likely related to our cave-dwelling, foraging-for-food ancestors. In times when food was scarce, we needed to "freshen our palates" to make sure we consumed a variety of foods available in nature, including a multitude of proteins, carbohydrates, and fats.

That's why we all get bored with an eating plan that focuses heavily on one of the big three nutrients (proteins, carbohydrates, fats), and restricts others—to the point that we can't stick with the plan. I've had so many patients tell me they haven't had bread in so long, they wanted to "gnaw the leg off a table," or that if they had one more piece of chicken they would "grow wings and fly away."

In your own toolbox, it's a good idea to keep a list of foods you consume regularly, to maintain structure and consistency (not too much temptation), and when it gets boring, switch gears to another food list.

### Sally's Story
## Help! I Love Bread!

Sally told me she felt doomed to weight-loss failure because of a life-long love affair with bread. She acknowledged that if she could only stay away from bread, she could stay on track with her weight-loss plan. Sally dropped bread cold turkey every time she went on a weight-loss plan. "Carbs are bad for me," she said, and noted that when she stayed away from bread and grains, she lost weight at the pace of about 3 pounds a week, for about a month. Then her plan stalled. After six to eight weeks on a no-grain plan, Sally jokingly told me, "I'd kill for a piece of bread." Feeling that she was failing, Sally would typically give up and go back to her old habits. That negative cycle was about to stop.

Sally agreed to face her sabotage of the all-or-nothing approach when it came to bread. When she agreed to limit—not eliminate—her intake of breads and starches, the overwhelming deprivation she felt when bread-free disappeared, and Sally began to feel more in control when choosing carbohydrates. When she understood that limiting starchy carbohydrates resulted in faster weight loss only because of the immediate water-loss features of low-carbohydrate eating, she agreed to be more patient in her expectations and aim for slower, steadier loss, with less frustration. Sally selected several starchy carbohydrates for her favorites list and consumed two or three servings a day. For Sally, these were reduced-calorie 100 percent whole wheat bread, 100-calorie whole wheat Thomas's English muffins, and 100-calorie whole wheat Weight Watchers pita. By limiting her choices to whole grain, portion-controlled bread products, Sally did not feel deprived. She also agreed to try a small baked potato to replace bread at dinner and was surprised to see how well it worked for her. While her intake of fruits and veggies remained high (she loved that water/fiber combination, which kept her feeling fuller longer), Sally had now figured out how to include some bread in her daily eating plan and still lose weight. She lost 7 pounds in the first month, a slower pace than when starch-free, but Sally felt confident that she could maintain her eating without feeling deprived. She was right. At the end of four months, she had lost 22 pounds. Bread was no longer the enemy. She agreed with my motto: "There are no bad foods, just bad portions."

---

# 10. Focus on Foods That Keep You Full

It's a biological fact: lean protein and high-fiber foods keep you fuller longer. What's more, water is a zero calorie diluter that provides extra volume (fills you up) without additional calories. Even air (think air-popped popcorn and seltzer) can plump up the food volume to keep you fuller longer. Isn't that the answer to the unspoken concern everyone struggles with when calorie cutbacks are a necessary part of weight loss? *We don't want to feel hungry.* While there are no promises in this department, the Real You eating plan provides a four-point foundation for basic eating satisfaction.

## 1. Lean Proteins: Animal and Vegetable

Long chains of amino acids (twenty-six different kinds) form different proteins for our bodies. While proteins support new muscle growth and development and are the precursors for production of several brain neurotransmitters, protein is also an important contributor to generating a strong satiety response when we eat. Protein foods provide value-added contentment, compared to equivalent amounts and calories of carbohydrate foods. Translated into calories, you'll tend to eat fewer calories and be more satisfied when you choose lean proteins. In nature, animal proteins are joined with fat (the artery-clogging type, if it's a beef product), and that's a choice to actively limit. When it comes to proteins, your toolbox should contain ultimate lean and super-lean choices. Anything else should be in the occasional indulgence department and saved for a special occasion.

How much protein do you need? Assuming you have no special health issues (especially kidney or liver disease), a good rule of thumb is to take your current weight and divide it in half—that's the number of daily protein grams to consume. If you weigh 140 pounds, aim for at least 70 grams of protein a day; at 180 pounds, about 90 grams of protein.

Check out the best proteins for your daily intake below.

### Ultimate Lean Proteins

Skinless white meat chicken or turkey breast
Fish fillet—all white fish (sole, haddock)
Shellfish (scallops, shrimps)
Ostrich
Water-packed solid white tuna
Egg whites
Egg substitutes
Fat-free hot dogs
Fat-free bologna

### Superior Lean Proteins

Dark meat chicken or turkey
Oily fish (salmon, trout, mackerel)
Canadian bacon
Whole eggs (limit 2 per day)
Flank steak
Top round beef
Ground sirloin
Beef cuts that must be marinated or stewed
Veal roast
Venison
Buffalo/Bison
Pork tenderloin
Low-fat hot dogs
Low-fat luncheon meat (ham, turkey pastrami)
Gefilte fish
Reduced-fat firm tofu

Soy burgers

Vegetable (black bean) burgers

### Double-Duty Proteins (containing calcium)

Milk, fat-free, 1 percent, or super-skim

Cottage cheese, fat-free, 1 percent or 2 percent, calcium-fortified

Cheese, single slices, fat-free or 2 percent (all brands)

Mozzarella cheese sticks, part-skim (all brands)

Yogurt, fat-free or low-fat plain (all brands)

Fruited yogurt, fat-free or low-fat with low-calorie sweetener (all brands)

Greek-style yogurt, fat-free plain (all brands)

Laughing Cow Light wedges or cubes

Mini Bonbel low-fat rounds

Soy milk plus calcium, fat-free

Here's another way to match up and compare your protein choices. It's a listing of foods and serving size, along with the grams of proteins and calorie counts.

| Food/Serving Size | Grams of Protein | Calories |
| --- | --- | --- |
| Fish—fresh, frozen, canned (4 ounces) | 28 | 160 |
| Meat—lean beef, veal, pork (4 ounces) | 28 | 225 |
| Poultry, skinless (4 ounces) | 28 | 160 |
| Calorie-controlled dinners (most brands have extra protein) | 18 to 30 | 250 to 400 |
| Soy burger (10 ounces) | 15 | 100 |
| Greek-style yogurt, nonfat, plain (8 ounces) | 16 | 120 |
| Yogurt, nonfat, sugar-free (8 ounces) | 8 | 100 |
| Egg, one whole large | 7 | 75 |
| Egg substitute (1/4 cup) | 5 | 25 |
| Soy nuts (1 ounce, about 30 nuts) | 12 | 120 |
| Tree nuts (1 ounce, about 25 nuts) | 6 | 160 |
| Peanut butter (1 tablespoon) | 4 | 100 |
| Skim milk (8 ounces) | 8 | 90 |
| Soy milk, fat-free (8 ounces) | 8 | 90 |
| Tofu (4 ounces) | 7 | 75 |

## 2. Carbohydrates: Fruits and Vegetables

Carbohydrates are nature's preferred energy source. Your metabolic pathways rely on carbohydrates as the basic building blocks of energy production. While our bodies know how to handle all carbohydrates, it's important from the weight-management viewpoint to consume carbohydrates that *don't* add a lot of extra calories due to hidden fats and extra sugars. The easiest way to avoid this problem is to limit processed foods. Seek out carbohydrates the way nature made them: an apple, not applesauce or apple juice; or brown rice, instead of white rice.

Fruits and vegetables are the perfect foods when it comes to losing weight. They are jammed with the two best possible calorie diluters: fiber and water, so you can eat a lot of volume for very few calories. And more volume equates to more fullness. You can thank the fiber for that. Fiber helps provide a feeling of fullness because it expands (with water) in your stomach like a sponge. It also helps to slow the rate of stomach emptying, and with more food remaining in your stomach for a longer time, you'll continue to feel content.

You can eat all vegetables as often as you like, except corn and peas, which fall in the starchy carbohydrate, low-water category (see "Fiber-Rich Starchy Carbohydrates" below). Feast while you're filling up on asparagus, bok choy, Brussels sprouts, broccoli, cabbage, carrots, celery, cauliflower, Chinese cabbage, cucumbers, eggplant, green beans, hot peppers, leeks, lettuce and other raw greens, kale, mushrooms, onions, parsnips, tomatoes, sweet peppers, yellow squash, and zucchini—just to name a few.

Fruits are nature's candy, and if you maximize your consumption of fresh fruits and limit the dried varieties (you want to keep that water in to bulk up the fruit), you'll satisfy your sweet tooth several times a day. Enjoy apples, apricots, berries, bananas, cherries, grapes, grapefruit, kiwi, lemons, limes, mango, melons, nectarines, oranges, peaches, pears, pineapple, plums, tangerines, and many more. Try frozen fruits right from the freezer.

## 3. Fiber-Rich Starchy Carbohydrates: Whole Grains

Starchy carbohydrates are everyone's favorites—and they should be part of any eating plan. It's the first place deprivation sets in when you try to cut them out altogether. When you stick with the fiber-rich varieties, you'll be able to consume a smaller portion and feel a lot fuller. While there's little water in the starchy carbohydrate group, the extra fiber alone helps promote fullness. When you choose processed grains—white flour products—they're not bad for you, it's just that you're likely to eat a lot more at one time, because nature's fullness secret has been stripped away. So you eat and eat—wondering why it takes so much more food to get to a point of satisfaction. While the texture of whole grains is somewhat chewier, the trade-off of a quicker feeling of fullness far outweighs any sensory adjustment. When you've been eating whole grains for about two weeks, you'll start wondering how you ever ate fluffy white flour products for so long. The robust and complex taste of whole grains is appreciated the more you eat it.

Vegetables that contain starchy carbohydrates include corn, beans (lima, pinto, kidney, cannellini, navy, black, chickpeas), sweet potatoes, and white potatoes. For grains, look for brown rice and whole wheat couscous, among others. For pasta, try flax or whole wheat varieties. Breads with a high fiber content include 100 percent whole wheat bread (light, regular, thin sliced), whole wheat tortillas, whole wheat matzoh, and whole wheat pita (try Weight Watchers), 100-calorie 100 percent whole wheat deli-thin rolls (try Arnold and Pepperidge Farm), and high-fiber 100-calorie English muffins (Thomas's and Weight Watchers make these).

There's a large variety of packaged foods with a high fiber content, such as microwave popcorn, Wheat Thins, Triscuit Thin Crisps, Kashi TLC single-serve crackers, Vitamuffin VitaTops, Barbara's Puffin Cereal, Fiber One cereal, Kashi Good Friends Cereal, Special K fiber-rich waffles, and several brands of instant or slow-cook oatmeal.

Of course, starchy carbohydrates contain the fiber, but not the *water*, of fruits and vegetables. That's why fruits and vegetables can be consumed in larger volumes, because that extra water greatly dilutes the calories. Be mindful of your portion sizes with starchy carbs.

Now that you understand the fiber basics, you can better choose the foods that work for you, to increase your daily fiber intake to at least

20 grams a day. It's also important to include both types of fiber found in foods, called "soluble" (related to blood cholesterol levels) and "insoluble" (related to regularity and digestive health).

*Soluble fiber* (dissolves in water): found in oats and oat bran, beans, fruits and vegetables.

*Insoluble fiber* (does not dissolve in water): found in wheat and corn bran, whole grains, fruits and vegetables.

When choosing fiber-rich foods, it's important to know both the serving size and the amount of fiber per serving. Below is a list to get you started. Remember, you're aiming for no less than 20 grams a day, with an upper limit of about 35 grams daily. If you're below 20 grams a day, increase your intake *slowly* to avoid stomach cramping and bowel disturbances. Plus, when you increase your fiber intake, you need to add fluid. Add at least one 8 ounce glass of water daily for every 5 grams of fiber you add to your diet, to ensure digestive balance. All that fiber needs liquid to keep it moving.

As you plan your fiber intake, remember these helpful hints:

- Aim for a minimum of 20 to 25 grams of fiber daily.
- A food with 3 grams of fiber per serving is a "good" source.
- A food with 5 grams (or more) of fiber per serving is a "high fiber" source.
- Increase your fiber intake gradually, by 5 or 6 grams per week.
- Increase your water intake when consuming more fiber. For every 5 grams of fiber added, increase your fluid intake by 8 to 10 ounces.
- Don't exceed 35 grams of fiber daily.
- Choose both insoluble- and soluble-fiber foods (fruits and veggies have both).
- Wash fruits thoroughly and eat the peel, for optimal fiber intake.
- Choose whole grain products; read labels for whole wheat as the first ingredient.
- Substitute canned beans for meat or chicken in a recipe; add a can to any soup or main dish for extra fiber.

Here's some help to raise your fiber awareness.

| Food/Serving Size | Grams of Fiber |
|---|---|
| *Fruits* | |
| Berries (1 cup) | 8 |
| Pear (medium) with skin | 5 |
| Apple (medium) with skin | 4 |
| Banana (medium) | 3 |
| Orange | 3 |
| Nectarine with skin | 3 |
| Peach with skin | 3 |
| Grapefruit ($1/2$) | 2 |
| Raisins ($1/4$ cup) | 2 |
| Plum (1 small) | 1 |
| Apricot | 1 |
| | |
| *Vegetables* | |
| Broccoli, 1 cup cooked | 6 |
| White potato, with skin (medium) | 5 |
| Sweet potato, with skin (medium) | 4 |
| Green peas, cooked ($1/2$ cup) | 4 |
| Corn, 1 cup (or 1 ear) | 4 |
| Winter squash ($1/2$ cup) cooked | 4 |
| Brussels sprouts ($1/2$ cup) cooked | 3 |
| Romaine lettuce, 3 cups fresh | 2 |
| Raw carrot, 1 medium | 2 |
| Raw cabbage, 1 cup | 2 |
| Spinach, raw, 1 cup | 1 |
| Tomato, 1 medium | 1 |
| | |
| *Dried Beans and Peas* | |
| Lentils, cooked ($1/2$ cup) | 8 |
| Split peas, cooked ($1/2$ cup) | 8 |
| Black-eyed peas, cooked ($1/2$ cup) | 6 |
| Baked beans, canned ($1/2$ cup) | 6 |
| Kidney, navy, pinto beans, cooked ($1/2$ cup) | 4 |

### Nuts and Seeds

| | |
|---|---|
| Almonds (1 ounce, about 24) | 4 |
| Peanuts, dry roasted (1 ounce, about 30) | 3 |
| Walnuts (1 ounce, about 20) | 3 |
| Peanut butter (2 tablespoons) | 2 |
| Sesame seeds (1 tablespoon) | 1 |

### Some Fiber-Fortified Foods

| | |
|---|---|
| Fiber One Honey Cluster Flakes (1 cup) | 13 |
| All-Bran (1/2 cup) | 9 |
| Fiber One Chewy Snack Bar | 6 |
| Weight Control oatmeal (1 packet) | 5 |
| Orange juice, calcium-fortified (8 ounces) | 5 |
| Fiber One yogurt (4 ounces) | 10 |

## 4. Smart Fats: Small Amounts of Heart-Healthy Sources

Fat is the macronutrient we love to hate. Many people wrongly think that if you eat fat, you'll become fat. While it's true that fat has twice the calories of the same portion of carbs or protein, a little fat goes a long way and is a very powerful tool when used properly. Here's how to do it.

Don't eliminate fat—it's quite important for hunger and fullness regulation. Fat slows the rate of stomach emptying, no matter what else is in your stomach. With your stomach holding food for a longer period of time, you stay satisfied. Fat is also amazingly palatable and tasty, and can enhance the flavor of most foods. Now the downside. Large amounts of fat are hidden in many foods, particularly in processed ones. If you're not a mindful eater, it's easy to eat way too much fat. For your BEAM Box, when you think "fat," I want you to think of three things: (1) choosing heart-healthy plant fats; (2) downsizing from full-fat to low-fat foods (nonfat is *not* always the right choice); and (3) limit portion size.

*Full fats:* Portion awareness is essential with these high-flavor-intensity foods.

- Avocados
- Tree nuts: almonds, cashews, pistachios, walnuts, hazelnuts
- Oils: olive, canola, safflower, sunflower, corn, sesame, flaxseed
- Peanuts

- Peanut butter (creamy or chunky) or almond butter
- Olives

*Fat substitutes:* Try these to reduce full-fat calories when you cook.

- Oil sprays: all flavors (for pans)
- Butter sprays: all brands (topping for vegetables, grains)
- Z-Trim: for baking

*Low-calorie fats* (all trans-fat-free): These are usually described as "light" or "reduced-fat." I'm not generally a fan of fat-free products — the removal of all fat takes away most of the taste, and often more calories are wasted by adding a larger portion, and more calories, to seek more taste. Fat-free products can be a caloric disaster waiting to happen. It's your choice if you want to use them, but be sure to monitor your portions carefully. Refer back to "Read Food Labels" on pages 57–59 for definitions of "light" and "fat-free" products.

- Light margarine
- Light butter
- Balada (reduced-fat butter)
- Light (or fat-free) salad dressing
- Light (or fat-free) cream cheese
- Light (or fat-free) mayonnaise

## 11. Always Have a Plan B

Having an alternate plan is the thinking person's tool for staying one step ahead. While the perfect-world food choices are your goal, your mind-set should always be to *do your best* to follow through with your original eating plan. When you are not able to follow through for some reason, you should be ready to adapt to whatever life has thrown your way. It's what I call the "Plan B approach." What if you've overslept and there's no time for breakfast? What if your favorite salad place in the airport is closed? What if you were too busy to go to the supermarket and there's nothing to eat at home?

To prevent a total collapse of your eating plan, always assume there will be times when you are stuck and will need a Plan B. The "B" stands for "backup." That's where meal replacements can fit in for everyone.

Carry along some nonperishable foods when you travel, something that, when combined with other foods, serves as a complete meal. That way, you'll always be sure to have a choice that keeps you on track. Keep some frozen calorie-controlled entrées in the freezer at home for times when you just can't get to the store or are simply too tired to cook.

## Plan B Foods

- Protein bars as a snack (100 calories) or a meal replacement (200–250 calories)
- Individual bags of nuts (pistachios, almonds, mixed nuts) (100–200 calories)
- 100-calorie pack raisins, dried cranberries, or mixed dried fruits

### Frank's Story
### I'm Always on the Road

As Frank explained to me, "I know what to do, but I'm always on the road, and I get off track." Whether he was at an airport, arriving late at a hotel when the restaurant was closed, or facing a handful of other situations, Frank often found himself hungry and without a healthy food option. He skipped meals and fell into the negative cycle of getting over-hungry and then overeating at the next meal. Frank loved his job, but he bemoaned his lifestyle and eating patterns and wanted to make a change. He'd been 35 pounds lighter nearly twenty years ago, when he was twenty-eight. Now, at age forty-eight, he wanted to lose about 20 pounds, and he wasn't in a hurry. He wanted to do it the right way and change his erratic eating. The solution for Frank was to develop his Plan B and assume that he'd always need to have a backup plan. He agreed that his good intentions of somehow finding some healthy foods when he needed them involved a bit of magical thinking and that he would need to carry some supplies with him, to stay on track.

We developed a plan where Frank would keep some nonperishable foods in his briefcase, to supplement his eating on the road, or even replace a meal, when needed, to fix the habit of meal skipping. He carried a combination of meal replacement bars (200–250 calories), snack bars (100 calories), and single-serve packs of almonds (100 calories). It started with breakfast. At the airport or on the road, Frank could always find a coffeehouse, but instead of coffee and a pastry, he chose a medium latte with skim milk. Or he had the option of a black coffee with one of his meal replacement bars. Frank learned to utilize the meal replacement bar when he was out of choices, particularly at the airport. He found that he could always find some fresh fruit, usually a banana, for easy eating. It also worked on airplanes. In anticipation of a client dinner meeting, Frank would have a package of nuts on the flight, along with a diet soda, which would help him transition to dinner.

After a little practice, Frank learned how he could make prepackaged and calorie-controlled foods work for him. He gained a sense of confidence, knowing that he had a backup plan for food when he needed it. It took him about four months to lose 15 pounds, and he is happy with his progress. Frank found a backup plan that worked for him when good intentions were not enough to keep him on track.

## 12. Use Meal Replacements

Meal replacements are a real plus for built-in calorie control. If you look at meal replacements as a tool to help keep you on track for times when you haven't preplanned, or are on the go, they are a food blessing. (One note of caution: if you regularly eat meal replacements because you are "afraid" of overeating on real food, meal replacements are not a positive tool for you. Go back to chapter 3 to address your food control issues.)

I'm not just talking about bars and shakes. Meal replacements are anything you can consume that is already preportioned and ready to eat—and you can eat the whole thing. Often packed with extra protein and fiber for greater satiety, meal replacements can also include calorie-controlled fresh or frozen meals that you buy at the supermarket, or even low-sugar, high-fiber, high-protein cereals mixed with some skim or low-fat milk. While it's economical to select "do-it-yourself" meal replacements, you can also pay much more to use a monthly commercial meal service. While this option can be a big boost for many people, those of you seeking greater value can choose from a variety of meals, shakes, and bars from your local market that can be rotated into your daily eating plan or replace it altogether for the first two weeks of your effort. Add unlimited fruits and vegetables from the master list, and you're on your way. Make sure you drink noncalorie and low-calorie fluids all day, letting thirst be your guide.

I look at this array of products as a way to jump-start your effort, with easy portion and calorie control at the start of a new effort. For most people, even replacing one meal a day can be a help. It takes the pressure off of making the right choice. Make sure you read the labels—check out the grams of protein (higher helps keep you satisfied longer) and total calories per bar (not just the serving).

While many bars *look* the same, the only way to know their nutrient content is to read the label. First, check the total calorie content of the bar to see if this falls in the range of a meal replacement or a snack. A good rule of thumb is to think of a snack as about 100 calories, and a meal as about 200 to 275 calories. Next, check the protein content. You'll want a meal replacement with 15 to 20 grams per bar. Look for snack bars with around 5 grams of protein (they're smaller, after all). Check out the sugar and fat content, and as a general rule, keep the sugars below 15 grams and the fat below 8 grams per bar.

Guidelines for bars and shakes: 150 to 220 calories, 15 to 25 grams protein

Guideline for fresh and frozen meals: 200 to 350 calories, 25 to 35 grams protein

## 13. Positive Snacking

It takes about 100 to 150 calories to satisfy between-meal hunger for most people. For some, even a 50-calorie snack is effective. The optimal choice is a snack that mixes at least two of the three macronutrients: protein, fiber-rich carbohydrate, and a small amount of fat. Some of the best choices are no-brainers, and are found in the 100-calorie snack pack aisle. When you're at home looking for a snack, think about the kind of food you really want. Decide if it's texture or flavor that you really seek. You'll spend a lot less time rummaging around your cabinets until you finally find the right taste. Do it up front, and your choice is more direct. The most common cravings are listed below.

You'll also be able to separate biological hunger from psychological hunger after a snack of about 100 calories. If you're feeling more content, it's biological hunger. If the snack fuels your hunger and triggers more eating, it's likely head hunger (see chapter 3).

**Most Common Taste and Texture Cravings**

Sweet and Creamy
Sweet and Chewy
Chocolate
Sweet and Crunchy
Salty and Crunchy
Salty and Chewy

# 14. Master Restaurant Eating

Often leaving our comfort zone of structure derails our eating plan. It's a mental battle to stay on track—and make your dining experience enjoyable and controlled, not stressful and full of deprivation. A patient once proudly told me that a friend asked her on one occasion where she wanted to dine out for dinner, saying that since she was on a diet, she probably couldn't eat at many places. My patient responded to her friend: "I can find something in *any* place we go." Now that is a liberating and empowering statement. It's all about making the right choice, and having the confidence that you can remain in control. No matter what type of restaurant you prefer, your eating strategy remains the same. By using the following restaurant mini-tools, you'll be able to socialize and control your eating, and feel satisfied without deprivation:

- Read the menu carefully and know what's in a dish.
- Order appetizers or small plates.
- Start off with a clear soup or plain mixed green salad.
- Order a clear soup or appetizer, and share a main dish.
- Ask for the salad dressing, sauce, and syrup on the side.

- Ask for a main dish to be steamed, baked, or broiled, without added fats.
- Remember the customer is always right; ask for exactly what you want.
- Have the bread basket removed from the table.
- Don't waste calories on liquids.
- Avoid fried foods, and substitute baked items.
- Order double vegetables with your entrée, and skip the starch.
- Share a dessert with at least one other person.
- Ask for milk instead of cream in your after-dinner coffee.

Here are a few of my favorite restaurant choices in four popular cuisines. You can mix and match (and share!) your own combinations.

### Asian Cuisine

*Appetizers:* hot and sour soup; egg drop soup, ginger salad (dressing on the side)

*Main dishes:* steamed shrimp and mixed vegetables (garlic sauce on the side); mu shu chicken (limit of one pancake); steamed tofu and mixed vegetables (brown sauce on the side)

*Sides:* extra order of vegetables; brown rice

*Desserts:* fortune or almond cookie (1)

### Italian Cuisine

*Appetizers:* minestrone soup; mixed green salad (dressing on the side)

*Main dishes:* grilled chicken or veal; meatballs; grilled fish

*Sides:* pasta with red sauce; steamed broccoli rabe or other green vegetable

*Desserts:* biscotti (1); fresh berries; cappuccino

(Note: Remove the breadbasket if it's a problem, or try eating only the crust of the bread, leaving the doughy middle.)

### Continental/New American

*Appetizers:* non-cream-based soup; salad (dressing on the side)

*Main dishes:* baked or broiled chicken, fish, or lean beef

*Sides:* baked or sweet potato; couscous; brown rice; steamed vegetables

*Desserts:* mixed berries (can add flavored liqueur); fruit tart (eat fruit, leave pastry)

## Diner/Family Restaurant

*Breakfast:* eggs/egg whites (poached or scrambled); vegetable omelet; rye or whole wheat toast; Canadian bacon; fresh fruit; oatmeal

*Lunch:* main dish salad with dressing on the side; sandwich on whole wheat bread with lettuce and tomato (take off one slice of bread, and use lettuce as top); water-packed tuna with greens; tomato or vegetable soup

*Dinner:* baked or broiled chicken or fish; portobello mushroom burger; baked potato; grilled or steamed vegetables

*Dessert:* Fresh fruit; baked apple

## Fast Food Restaurant

*Main dishes:* chicken fajita (skip the sour cream); bean burrito; kid's meal (small burger, small fries, diet soda or water); grilled chicken sandwich; chili; baked potato (skip the cheese sauce and ask for salsa)

## 15. Control Special Occasion Eating

The best time to give yourself permission to indulge smartly is for an occasion that is special to you. It will only work if you are honest with yourself and are monitoring your eating most days and indulge only *occasionally.* For a major family holiday or get-together, a wedding, or a reunion, it's really okay to allow yourself some favorite indulgences and include some preplanned "off the track" eating. It's important to give yourself permission so you're not sneaking around and then feeling guilty when you eat the forbidden foods. Remember, there are no bad foods, just bad portions. You don't need to barter; you can allow yourself the treat of eating a small amount of anything you want. It's only one meal (or one day), and if you are committed to your Real You plan, and your BEAM Box is full of tools, you can readily have some special occasion eating days in a year.

*Lisa's Story*
## My Life Is Full of Eating Events

Lisa comes from a large, close-knit family, where, as she put it, "Food is definitely love." It wasn't just family holidays, but rather that almost every week there was a major eating event. In addition to their traditional extended family dinner on Sundays, it always seemed to be someone's birthday or anniversary, or some other reason to celebrate with a big dinner. Lisa found herself attending these events at least twice a week and being pressured by her family members to eat.

At twenty-three, Lisa was happy in her job as an elementary school teacher in her hometown school district. She lived in an apartment just a short drive from the neighborhood in which she grew up. While that provided a lot of joy in her life, Lisa felt she was locked into all these events where the family celebrated with food. Lisa's parents and extended family were "big people," as she put it. They were happy with their lives and did not see weight control as a priority. Lisa felt frustrated that she was being talked into eating with the idea that every family get-together was a special occasion. Lisa recognized that this was a major sabotage of her own efforts, and she needed some help. She'd gained about 30 pounds in the two years since she'd returned to her hometown and attributed much of it to these family dinners.

It was time for Lisa to make some changes. She agreed that a true special occasion warranted some indulgent eating, but that those occasions needed to be limited to about once a month. Lisa had an open conversation with her mother about her weight. While her mother did not necessarily agree with Lisa's weight-loss goals, she did agree to prepare some different foods for Lisa that would be compatible with her calorie-controlled eating plan. Lisa also volunteered to bring either a steamed vegetable dish or a bowl of cut-up fruit as her contribution to the meals.

Lisa understood that she could change only her own behavior, and that her mother derived great joy when cooking for her. To allow her mother to keep that joy, Lisa asked her mother to prepare some of her favorite foods for each gathering. Now no longer a passive participant in the menus, Lisa always found some good choices when she attended family dinners; and following her mother's lead, the other relatives learned to let Lisa eat what she preferred. Lisa found herself enjoying her family gatherings, since food was no longer the focus for her. She felt empowered now, as she could choose the event that she viewed as a "special occasion," and on those days she made some smart indulgences. Lisa had found the balance for herself and added the special tool to allow herself some indulgent eating, with boundaries, to refine her BEAM Box. She stopped her slowly creeping weight and lost 12 pounds in her first three months after making those family events a part of her regular eating pattern most of the time.

---

## 16. Learn to Face Liquid Calories and Alcohol

In the perfect drinking world, we would all prefer water, and we wouldn't have any other choices. Alas, in the real world, liquid calories are everywhere, and in such large portions! Liquid calories fall into that category of diet fantasy of "not counting"—like those calories we consume while standing up or on a special date. (I hope you appreciate my diet humor.) The beverage industry has gotten out of control—with size, with options, and with calories. The choices are endless, and label reading is a must-do. Most beverages now come in gigantic sizes and multiple colors (beware—not all clear drinks are calorie-free), and range from zero calories per serving to several hundred. Plus, some healthy, lower-calorie drinks have morphed into calorie sinkholes due to supersizing.

Alcohol can be the downfall of even the most structured weight-loss plan. It you would rather eat than consume alcohol calories, then go ahead and skip this section. If you're someone who would rather barter some alcohol calories, either daily or on the weekend, for a modest food exchange, it is possible to do so with some effort. The problem with alcoholic drinks is that it's often hard to find the calories per serving, and serving sizes vary enormously anyway. Beverage mixers come prepackaged and loaded with extra calories, while many restaurants offer fruit-based mixed drinks in gigantic souvenir glasses.

Why do we drink so many extra calories? Here's a biological truth: our bodies do not sense liquid calories very well. We do much better with solid foods when it comes to calorie consumption. Our bodies do not count 500 extra calories from liquids as they would from solid food. We tend to eat just as much during the day as if we hadn't had those fluids. Those calories you drink from every source, healthy or not, will add to your total daily calorie consumption and not add to your feeling of fullness. So just 500 extra calories a day from liquids can pack on 1 extra pound in a week.

### Eight Liquid Mini-Tools

- Water—sparkling or still—is always your best choice.
- When it comes to regular soda and juice, downsize your drink, and skip the free refills.
- Choose low-calorie sodas, juices, and flavored waters.
- Look for low-calorie powdered sachets to add to water.
- Dilute 100 percent juice with water or seltzer; one part juice to three parts water.
- Choose low-fat or nonfat dairy beverages.
- Order a small size from a coffeehouse or a smoothie bar.
- Read labels: "clear" and "healthy" don't always mean calorie-free.

### Eight Alcohol Mini-Tools

- Measure, don't eyeball, your serving.
- Choose light beer in a bottle for optimal portion control.
- Avoid fruit drinks and sugary mixed drinks.
- Mix spirits with seltzer, diet soda, or water.
- Replace regular tonic water with sugar-free (diet) tonic water.
- Use a smaller wine glass.
- Try a wine spritzer (half wine, half seltzer).
- Limit your consumption by alternating a tall glass of club soda with lime with each alcoholic drink.

# 17. Take Your Vitamins and Minerals

Taking a daily multiple vitamin is a must-do when cutting back on calories. It gives you good insurance that you're meeting all your vitamin and mineral requirements. But you don't have to spend extra money on organic vitamins or special formulations. Name brands and generics are both good choices. When it comes to vitamins, cost does not always indicate biological equivalency or guarantee a better product. Check with your doctor for any special needs relating to your personal medical condition, medications you take, or your age that might require additional supplementation with iron, B vitamins, or other compounds.

Some other things to remember:

• You'll want to stick with a vitamin/mineral supplement that provides 100 percent of the recommended daily allowance (RDA) in a single pill or capsule, plus a calcium supplement. Read the dose. Children's chewables and some others often need two or more doses to get the 100 percent RDA.

• If you think more is better when it comes to vitamins and minerals, beware! There are recommended upper limits, especially for calcium and fat-soluble vitamins. These are the ones retained by your body and not flushed out in your urine like the water-soluble ones. Check with your doctor or pharmacist for more information, not online with Dr. Google. Here are just a few examples:

| Vitamin/Mineral | 100% RDA/Upper Limit |
|---|---|
| Calcium* | 1,000 mg/2,500 mg |
| Iron** | 18 mcg/45 mcg |
| Vitamin A | 3,000 mg/10,000 mg |
| Vitamin D | 400 mg/2,000 mg |

\* Requirement varies from 1,000 to 1,500 mg/day

\*\* Iron supplementation to be avoided in men and postmenopausal women

Your daily foundation for vitamins and minerals should include:

• Vitamin/mineral supplement: 100% RDA (use iron-free for men and for women over fifty)

• Calcium supplement (500 to 1,000 mg) with vitamin D

You might also consider (check with your doctor):

- Vitamin D supplementation, 400 to 800 mg daily
- Fish oil capsules, 1,000 mg (active essential fatty acids) daily

Check with your doctor or pharmacist if you take prescription medication that requires more or less of specific vitamins and minerals.

In addition to your daily multivitamin, you will need a calcium supplement. With dairy product consumption severely declining around age ten, most women and men need this supplement to support adequate intake of about 1,000 mg per day. Is that a lot? Yes, it's about three servings every day. For most dieters, that's just not practical. Check out your own age group below. And don't be confused by all the supplements out there. More is not always better, especially when it comes to calcium. Take a cue from nature and look for about 500 mg per capsule (or pill or chew)—the amount in a large dairy serving. Vitamin D can enhance absorption, and most products contain 200 to 400 mg of added vitamin D. You can also just take a non-D calcium supplement along with your daily vitamin (which already contains vitamin D).

| Age | Calcium per Day |
| --- | --- |
| Up to 18 | 1,300 mg |
| 19 to 50 | 1,000 to 1,200 mg |
| 51+ | 1,200 to 1,500 mg |
| Special Needs (nursing/pregnant) | 1,200 to 1,500 mg |

While dairy products contain the most concentrated amounts of calcium per serving, you can also help meet your calcium needs with other fortified and nondairy foods. Here are some helpful calcium amounts. Aim to get at least 500 mg daily from foods, with any remaining deficits made up with a daily calcium supplement.

### Foods That Contain about 300 mg Calcium (30%) per Serving:

8 ounces milk (fat-free, low-fat, whole)

8 ounces yogurt (plain or fruit)

8 ounces soy milk

1/2 ounce natural cheese (Swiss, cheddar, pepper jack, mozzarella)

2 ounces processed American cheese

1/4 cup Parmesan cheese

$^1/_2$ cup ricotta cheese

$^1/_2$ cup calcium-fortified cottage cheese

1 cup calcium-fortified juice

## Foods That Contain about 200 mg Calcium (20%) per Serving:

3 ounces sardines (with bones)

3 ounces canned salmon (with bones)

1 cup calcium-fortified cereal

6 ounces calcium-fortified juice

## Foods That Contain about 150 mg Calcium (15%) per Serving:

4 ounces yogurt (plain or fruit)

4 ounces pudding

1 cup cottage cheese (unfortified)

$^1/_2$ cup low-fat tofu

$^1/_2$ cup cooked or 1 cup raw spinach

1 slice calcium-fortified bread

## Foods That Contain about 100 mg Calcium (10%) per Serving:

1 cup broccoli

1 cup canned beans

$^1/_4$ cup raw almonds

4 figs (fresh or dried)

1 ounce fat-free cream cheese

# 5

# Activity Tools
## Deciding How and When to Move

**You'll notice** I'm not calling these "exercise" tools, but "activity" tools. To me, there's a big difference. Over the past decade or two, as a nation we've become a lot less active. How did this happen? With advances in consumer technology reducing our activity, we now move a lot less during the day than we did a generation or two ago. It's just much easier to sit around. Think about it. We don't have to get up and change the TV channel (giant remote), or walk down the hall to give a coworker a message (e-mail), or even roll down the windows in our car (electric controls). For many people, exercise is just one more thing to add to an already overscheduled day. That's why I'm all for a return to the natural physical activity we can all include as part of everyday living.

The good news is that the vast majority of physically active people don't need a variety of special or expensive equipment, a trainer, or an army of helpers. While those can be a plus for some people, they're not essential. What physically active people do have is a commitment to moving more every day. It's what I call "activity of daily living," the foundation of an active lifestyle. A variety of solo and group activities with different types of intensity and duration can be added to support this activity base. The main goal is to sit less.

While we're all familiar with the food pyramid, far fewer of us know about the activity pyramid (page 95). There's a lot of confusion about what really counts as physical activity. Running? Weight lifting? Yoga? Isn't just walking good enough anymore? The answer to all of these questions is a resounding yes. When you understand the activity pyramid, you'll see that all kinds of activity are important—and fit together like a jigsaw puzzle. The Real You plan suggests a variety of physical activity tools you can pull out at any time. They are all important, and you'll want to choose several tools, to avoid activity boredom and burnout. Whether it's strength training, cardiovascular endurance, joint health, relaxation, or just the fun of movement, once you develop some physical activity tools, you'll optimize your rate of weight loss, as well as have some insurance toward keeping that weight off for good.

One more thing: while mental preparation is essential, *always* check with your doctor first (see chapter 6) to make sure you're physically prepared for the challenges of new or extended activity.

## Adding Up Daily Activity

Just 100 extra calories burned each day will translate into about 10 pounds lost by the end of a year. It's easier to do than you may think. Here's what a simple five minutes can do:

| In the House | Calories Used |
| --- | --- |
| Washing floors/Vacuuming | 25 |
| Dusting/Making beds | 15 |
| Cooking | 10 |
| Standing and writing your shopping list | 10 |

| In the Yard or in Town | Calories Used |
|---|---|
| Shoveling snow | 43 |
| Playing touch football | 42 |
| Playing tag | 38 |
| Playing tennis (doubles) | 35 |
| Bowling | 33 |
| Weeding | 30 |
| Planting | 25 |
| Golfing | 20 |
| Grocery shopping | 15 |

Take a look at the activity pyramid below for a better idea of how to mix and match activities in your life. Don't approach activity with an all or nothing mind-set. Your foundation should be built on increased "activity of daily living" and supported by a variety of other activities of your choosing. Depending on your own preferences (refer to "Your

**Activity Pyramid**

**As Little as Possible**

Sit watching TV, playing video games, or working on the computer

**2 to 3 Days per Week**

*Sports, Strength, Active Leisure*
swimming, lifting weights, gardening, yoga, pilates, tai chi, bowling, touch football

**3 to 5 Days per Week**

*Planned Aerobic/Cardio Activities*
jogging, running, biking, dancing, cardio DVDs, jumping rope, tennis, stair/elliptical machine, rowing, shoveling snow, hand-mowing the grass

**Every Day**

*Activity of Daily Living*
taking the stairs, parking far away and walking, washing the car, cleaning the house, grocery shopping, walking the dog, losing the TV remote, walking while talking on the phone

Physical Activity Temperament" on page 100), you'll be able to select additional activities that you enjoy and can sustain as important life-long tools.

When choosing your activities, there are three issues you will need to consider:

- *Duration*: How long and how often am I willing to do this?
- *Intensity*: How strenuous an effort do I want to make? Do I prefer a more vigorous effort in a shorter period of time, or do I want a more modest effort of longer duration?
- *Rate of Perceived Exertion (RPE)*: How do I pace myself for optimal health benefit, calorie utilization, and enjoyment? (See the chart on page 97 for some guidelines.) RPE is the newest way to gauge activity level and easier to measure than heart-rate alone. It helps you evaluate both duration and intensity of an activity. If you're just getting started, the RPE is the way to go. If you have a heart-rate monitor, add the RPE as a support to stay connected to your workouts.

## Using the RPE Scale

This easy, modified, 10-point RPE scale is one way to gauge your activity level. You do not need any special equipment to measure your exertion, because it is all based on your own personal assessment of how much you are exerting yourself. A rating of 2 is light, nonstrenuous activity. It might be a walk to get the morning paper. A rating of 9 is intense activity that cannot be sustained for more than a few minutes, such as a fast walk up a steep hill or a fast run down the street. (The time can increase as you become more highly conditioned.)

The beauty of the RPE scale is that there are no right answers. Some days you might be able to walk faster outside and tackle more hills, or set an exercise machine at greater resistance. Other days, you'll turn down the intensity and stay in a lighter exertion range. The most important thing is to listen to your body signals and adjust your activity to how you feel.

**Rate of Perceived Exertion**
- 0   At Rest—No exertion
- 2   Very Light
- 4   Light
- 6   Somewhat Hard
- 8   Very Hard
- 10  Maximal Exertion

Use this RPE scale as a guideline when selecting your physical activity tools. The RPE is a balance between intensity (how hard you work) and duration (how long you do it). Your goal is a mix of moderate activity (4 to 6 RPE)—think of walking and being able to talk comfortably—and more vigorous activity (7 to 9 RPE). At the more intense activity level, it will be hard to talk while moving. The first step is making a habit of activity—frequency is key. Moving every day—at different levels of the RPE scale—is the most important factor. Your long-term RPE goal has two parts: (1) at least 150 weekly minutes of activity in the 4 to 6 range (a brisk walk) and (2) a minimum of 90 extra minutes per week in the 7 to 9 range. When you have established a habit and reached a comfort level with 150 minutes per week, add 30 minutes three times a week of activity in the 7 to 9 range.

You can balance your RPE to fit your time and energy level. Think of the weekends as time to catch up on your activity. It's amazing how many people think that the weekends are off days for activity. For most people, it's a great time to pick up the pace. Take a look at how two busy people, with very different lifestyles, managed their activity goals using the weekly RPE approach. When you think about your activity in a *weekly* mode, it reduces a lot of mental pressure associated with regular activity.

## Lana's RPE Plan

Lana, a senior executive and the mother of two preschoolers, came to me with a specific problem. She always enjoyed being physically active, and while her time was limited, she wanted to do more than get more steps in her day. She struggled with finding the time to exercise regularly and still have enough time to spend with her daughters and her husband, also a busy professional. Lana's everyday activity was in the RPE 4 to 6 range — parking farther away and quickly walking to her destination, taking four flights of stairs at work instead of the elevator. A major step was to get her husband to watch the girls so she could fully commit to a regular more intense workout twice each week. Her husband agreed to spend time with the girls on Saturday mornings so Lana could go to a one-hour kickboxing class at the local community center, as well as Wednesday evenings, when Lana attended a water aerobics class at the local high school pool. Once or twice a week, Lana also put in an exercise walking DVD that she and her daughters enjoyed as a family activity. Lana found that the commitment of twice a week for her more intense activities for a limited time was workable. She could structure this time, know her daughters were enjoying time with their dad, and be mentally focused on herself. Her remaining activity was a combination of daily activity in the workplace and at home with her family.

### Lana's Weekly Activity Log

| Activity | Duration (RPE) |
|---|---|
| Cumulative walking | 140 min/week (4–6) |
| Water jogging | 60 min/week (8) |
| Kickboxing | 60 min/week (8–9) |
| Walking DVD | 30 min/week (4–6) |

#### Lana's Total Weekly Time
170 minutes/week at RPE 4–6
120 minutes/week at RPE 7–9

## Dave's RPE Plan

Dave's goals were similar to Lana's, but he was at a very different stage of life. He also was concerned that he had no time to devote to his activity regimen. Single, with a demanding job as a software engineer, Dave "was always working," as he said. He had trouble figuring out how to let go of his work and focus on some regular activity. His company had a gym, which Dave rejoined. He had belonged before, but never went, so he quit; but now he wanted to make his activity a priority. Dave's earlier mistake had been to listen to coworkers who always exercised in the early morning, to "get it out of the way." These guys, he said, were at the gym when it opened at 5 a.m., worked out, showered, and were hard at work by 8 a.m. Dave was a night owl, so this just didn't work for him. He agreed that he could not reliably take a break in the middle of the day, although he had tried to convince himself that a break would be a good stress reliever.

Dave's new plan was to devote regular time at the end of the day for intense RPE during the workweek, since he was glued to his desk for most of the time, and activity of daily living was not sufficient exercise for him. Dave made the gym part of his daily workweek. He went to the gym five days a week, and cross-trained on the elliptical or the treadmill at an incline for 30 minutes at an RPE of 6 to 8. He also lifted weights twice a week (after four introductory sessions from the trainer, to develop a plan to do on his own and to ensure correct form) for another thirty minutes at 7 to 9 RPE. Dave saved the weekends for leisurely walks with his girlfriend—a visit to a museum, the mall, or other "knocking around" activities, as he called them. Dave did well thinking of his physical activity as a weekly accumulation, and the balance of greater intensity during the week, with a more relaxed weekend, worked for him.

### Dave's Weekly Activity Log

| Activity | Duration (RPE) |
| --- | --- |
| Treadmill/Elliptical | 150 min/week (7–8) |
| Weight lifting | 60 min/week (7–9) |
| Weekend walking | 120 min/week (4–6) |
| Weekday walking | 50 min/week (4–6) |

### Dave's Total Weekly Time

170 min/week at RPE 4–6
210 min/week at RPE 7–9

# Your Physical Activity Temperament

Your first tool is an understanding of your activity temperament. The only way you'll stick with any activity is if you enjoy it. Let's face it— there are some activities you don't like and you'll never like, and others that you'll embrace. I'm a big advocate of trying a new activity, but some things you just can't force. Check out these different activity personalities, and think about which one best fits your profile. Then see how these match up to the variety of activities on the exercise pyramid. Remember, there is no perfect activity; picking and choosing wisely is the key to helping you stay connected for life. The profiles range from the self-starting loner to the socially engaged team person. When taking the first step to adding any new activities, give some thought to what you naturally like to do.

**Your Activity Temperament**

- Loner
- One Partner
- Small Group
- Organized Team

*Sally's Story*
## I Can't Stick with an Exercise Plan

Sally came in to see me, knowing that she needed to increase her physical activity. She felt very guilty about her inability to stick with a variety of activities, so we discussed her activity temperament, a concept that Sally had never really thought about. She had always considered herself an outgoing, group-activity person and tended to select physical activities geared to that. She had tried a number of classes and always dropped out after a few sessions. She figured it was because the activity was "not for her." Even a walking group didn't seem to click. As an intensive care nurse in a busy hospital, Sally wanted to be more physically active, both for the short-term benefit as a stress reliever and the long-term health benefits. As we chatted, Sally acknowledged that she always felt a lot of pressure to "keep up with the group," whether it was a structured class or even the walking group. In fact, the group setting provided yet another opportunity for her to be competitive, which generated more stress for her.

In thinking this through, Sally agreed that she was happiest exercising by herself, enjoying her own private thoughts, some music, or a favorite TV show for company. She could work out at her own pace and not feel the need to keep up with anyone else. Sally was liberated after seeing that when it came to exercise, she was a solo exerciser and was best off going it alone. She purchased an elliptical machine for her apartment and used it daily while watching the evening news. Sally also purchased a Power Yoga DVD for strength training, which she did twice weekly in the privacy of her living room. More than a year later, Sally is still committed to her program and knows that when she needs a change, she'll look for solo activities. She's looking into purchasing a Wii Fit for herself for added stimulation. She understood that there was nothing wrong with her in wanting her regular physical activity to be solo. Now, she finds that group activities with friends, including walking, can be a social, enjoyable occasion, since the goal is no longer part of her regular regimen.

---

# Activity of Daily Living: Moving More Every Day

Move more, whenever you can. That is the foundation of activity of daily living. Stand instead of sit. Take the stairs instead of the escalator. Park farther away from your destination. No matter where you are, or what you're doing, think of ways to add some steps.

- Purchase a pedometer, as an easy way to track your activity. While the ultimate goal is 10,000 steps or more a day for both heart health and weight control, that's a challenge for most people just starting out.

Here's how to begin:

- Wear the pedometer for three days and write down your daily steps.
- Figure out the average number of steps you took each day, and make that your daily goal for the rest of the week.
- Each week after that, work on a goal of averaging 1,000 extra steps a day, at least three days that week.
- When you can master 1,000 extra steps a day most days, make that your new goal for daily steps.
- Work your way up to 10,000 steps a day—about 4 miles.

For example, if you walked 2,000 steps the first day, 2,500 steps the second day, and 3,000 steps the third day, your average daily steps for three days was 2,500. For the rest of the week, make 2,500 steps your daily goal. On three days of the next week, try to add 500 steps each day, to a total of 3,000 steps. Then work up to a goal of adding 1,000 steps every day—continuing to add steps each week until you are doing 10,000 steps a day.

The beauty of walking and using a pedometer is that there is no rush, no race. You can do this at your own pace—with just five minutes to spare, or thirty minutes. For every 2,500 steps you walk, you burn about 100 calories, and 10,000 steps is about 4 miles—or about 400 calories you don't even have to break a sweat over. *This is a powerful tool: you can lose 2 to 3 pounds a month—before you've even made a dent in your food intake!*

### *Emily's Story*
### I Can't Separate Physical Fatigue
### from Mental Fatigue

Emily already felt she had a very active day, and she did a lot of walking in her job as a pharmaceutical representative. Because she traveled a lot, both by car and plane, she often had no idea of her level of physical activity and sometimes couldn't tell if she was physically fatigued from being on the go or just mentally fatigued from the stress of the job. For Emily, the best tool to monitor this was a pedometer to keep track of her daily steps. It gave her a way to increase her activity in a structured way, and she could separate her mental fatigue from her physical fatigue. We set her daily step goal at 10,000 steps, as her activity of daily living was something she could do consistently. She had been taking around 7,500 steps on many days, and now she was able to make the consistent effort of those extra steps. She walked home from work—about 1 mile—which gave her extra steps and burned about 100 extra calories, Her daily walk home took only another twenty minutes at the end of the day, and it had the added bonus of being a great stress reliever. All Emily needed was a way to monitor her activity. The pedometer did the trick.

---

## *Paula's Story*
## I Want to Do More Than Walk

Paula told me she had never been a regular exerciser, and she agreed that this was part of the reason she had struggled with her weight since her teens. "I'm just not athletic," she told me. Paula had just celebrated her fortieth birthday, and her gynecologist had recently mentioned that her weight had gone up about 5 pounds in the past year. This mother of two told me she wanted "to be around" for her children and to get into shape. She wanted to lose about 20 pounds. For the first time in her life, Paula agreed to make activity a regular part of her life. She agreed that she had a lot of tools in her BEAM Box, but not many of them in the way of exercise. She began with a pedometer and was doing well—she had reached 6,000 steps daily and was working toward 10,000 steps a day (within another month). Paula wanted to gain some strength, and she was interested in gaining some core strength and improving her balance. Paula noticed that she could not stand on one foot and put a sock on her other foot while standing. She just couldn't keep her balance.

Paula and I discussed some options to get started. As someone who wasn't very confident in her abilities, Paula needed to start with an activity that would build her sense of accomplishment. And that's where the Wii Fit came in. Paula mentioned that her sons loved their Wii Sports video games, and that she and her husband recently had bought the Wii Fit package to give the boys more physical activity. Paula became the newest family member to use the Wii Fit. Her sons set her up and helped her with the exercises. Using the fitness board, Paula was amazed at how well she did and felt a real sense of accomplishment. She became a regular user—about three times a week. Paula felt that her balance improved a great deal, her core (back and abdomen) felt stronger, and her posture was much improved.

Her regular activity was now a real boost to her energy level, and Paula felt more motivated to push herself in her daily walking. She reached her daily goal of 10,000 steps and sometimes exceeded this on the weekends. Her Wii Fit sessions were something she looked forward to. In two months, without modifying her diet, Paula lost 5 pounds. With her activity tools firmly in her BEAM Box, Paula is now contemplating some changes in her daily eating to increase her rate of weight loss. Now that exercise is a habit, she can focus more easily on other kinds of changes she is both willing and able to make.

## Aerobic Activity: Picking Up the Pace

Aerobic activity gets your heart rate up (safely) and burns more calories than gentler activity. On the RPE scale of 1 to 10 for effort, aerobic activity falls in the 6 to 9 range.

If you want to use your heart rate as your guide for the time and intensity of your exercise routine and don't have a monitor, all you need is this easy calculation to find your target rate. To measure your heart rate, place your index finger on the inside of your wrist and locate your pulse point (where you feel regular throbbing). Count each pulse for 30 seconds and then double that number to determine your heart rate. If you're interested in a more precise heart rate measurement, I recommend you purchase a simple heart-rate monitor instead of depending on your gym equipment. The numbers provided by exercise machines are estimates and not a reliable or consistent gauge of your heart rate.

To calculate your target heart rate, take the number 220 and subtract your age; then multiply that number by 0.7. The number you get is your target heart rate per minute, which you can sustain for as little as a few minutes to as long as thirty minutes or more, if you're willing and physically able. Here are a few examples:

**Age 30**
220 – 30 = 190
0.7 × 190 = 133, your target heart rate per minute.

**Age 40**
220 – 40 = 180
0.7 × 180 = 126, your target heart rate per minute.

**Age 50**
220 – 50 = 170
0.7 × 170 = 119, your target heart rate per minute.

Remember, as you get more fit, it takes more effort to raise your heart rate, which also increases the amount of effort you need to raise your RPE. Talk to an exercise physiologist or certified trainer when your fitness level begins to increase.

Not sure how to get started? Check with a friend or coworker or a family member about what aerobic activities they do. Ask to join in, or ask how to find other people who are at your starting skill level. It's always easier to start a new activity with others who are newbies as well.

For those of you who just want an easy and economical way to get moving, I'd suggest a simple walking or walking/running plan. You don't need special training or equipment, just a pair of good walking shoes. A pedometer allows you to keep track of your progress and provides evidence of your daily and weekly progress. This is a big help in setting realistic activity goals. You can also incorporate interval training (see page 112), both to increase your exercise efficiency and to shake up your routine by varying your pace from a stroll (100 steps a minute, or about 3 miles per hour) to a brisk walk (about 150 steps a minute, or about 4 miles per hour).

## The Real You Four-Week Walking Plan

Before you start:

- Stand up straight (not rigid and stiff).
- Walk with your head up, looking straight ahead
- Remember to take long, comfortable strides.
- Keep your arms relaxed at your sides.
- Keep your RPE between 4 and 6.
- Walk a minimum of four days per week.

  *Week 1:* 20 minutes/day
     Walk 5 minutes; walk 10 minutes *briskly*; walk 5 minutes
  *Week 2:* 25 minutes/day
     Walk 5 minutes; walk 15 minutes *briskly*; walk 5 minutes
  *Week 3:* 30 minutes/day
     Walk 5 minutes; walk 20 minutes *briskly*, walk 5 minutes
  *Week 4:* 35 minutes/day
     Walk 5 minutes; walk 25 minutes *briskly*; walk 5 minutes

Your next step: If you love your walking routine, just stick with it. Consistency is key. No need to push ahead, if you're happy. But if you're looking for a little more, try some interval training by mixing up brisk walking with some slow running. Here's how.

## The Real You Four-Week Walk/Run Plan

Before you start:

- Make sure you can walk 30 minutes at a brisk pace (an RPE between 4 and 6).
- Walk with your head up, looking straight ahead.
- Remember to take long, comfortable strides.
- Keep your arms relaxed at your sides.
- For the running part of your plan, aim for an RPE between 7 and 9.
  *Week 1:* 30 minutes/day

     Walk 5 minutes; walk 5 minutes briskly; alternate brisk walking with slow running for 10 minutes (aim for slow running intervals of 1 to 2 minutes); walk 5 minutes.

*Week 2*: 35 minutes/day

Walk 5 minutes; walk 10 minutes *briskly*; alternate brisk walking with slow running for 15 minutes (aim for slow running intervals of 1 to 2 minutes); walk 5 minutes.

*Week 3*: 35 minutes/day

Walk 5 minutes; walk briskly for 5 minutes; alternate brisk walking with slow running for 20 minutes (aim for slow running intervals of 2 to 3 minutes); walk 5 minutes.

*Week 4*: 35 minutes/day

Walk 10 minutes briskly; alternate brisk walking with slow running for 20 minutes (aim for slow running intervals of 3–4 minutes); walk 5 minutes.

Still looking for more? If you enjoy the balance of walking and running, and you feel great, stick with this as your final goal for now. If you're able to slow run for at least 15 minutes and you like the feel of running, you might want to further challenge yourself and pursue a running plan, and perhaps train for races and be on your way toward being a more serious runner. Training for a 5K or 10K race in your area is a good way to start.

# Strength Training

Strength training, or lifting weights, is an important component of weight management. Most of us can't keep up our muscle strength solely with the activities of daily living—things like lifting grocery bags, lifting our children, and lugging suitcases. With less use, we do lose muscle mass every decade, and it's something that requires effort to sustain, for weight management and for overall health. Metabolically, muscle has twice the activity of fat, meaning you use twice as many calories to keep muscle tissue working in the body, compared to fat tissue. That is a major factor in avoiding weight creep year after year. Our metabolism naturally slows by about 5 percent each decade after age thirty. Translated into calories, that's about 100 or so calories less every day just to stay even and not gain weight.

There's not much you can do to fool Mother Nature, but increasing muscle mass (while decreasing body fat at the same time, nature's perfect yin and yang) can fight this off. You'll want to balance your upper-body and lower-body strength and focus on more than one or two areas of particular interest. All muscle groups are important. Plus, having more muscle mass is good for your bone health, as this provides extra weight-bearing exercise—just carrying yourself around uses more energy and is a big plus for both burning calories and supporting bone density.

An important component of strength training involves strengthening your body core. Your core is the area between the shoulders and hips, also known as your trunk. A lot of recent emphasis from health and fitness professionals is on development of core strength as the central focus of the body. Strengthening your back muscles and abdominal muscles is essential to developing a strong core.

Core strength can be increased easily by being mindful of your posture. Your mom was right—stand up straight! Standing tall forces you to keep your abdominal muscles contracted and your back erect, improving core muscle tone. When you are ready to move on to specific core-strengthening exercises, you can refer to the list on the next page to get you started.

A variety of balance activities and exercises can also help your core. Try sitting on an exercise ball instead of a chair. You will need to use your core muscles to maintain your balance, which will give them a good workout. You can also try classes using exercise balls or rent a DVD focusing on your core. Even the Wii Fit has some exercises to strengthen these muscles.

Activities such as yoga, Pilates, tai chi, and others are great for developing and maintaining core strength (plus they do double duty with relaxation—see the section on mind-body below).

The twelve exercises below will help get you started with strength training. You can use free weights or use your body weight as resistance. If you plan on using free weights (for hands or ankles) or a weighted vest, you should consult a professional to determine proper form and the best starting weight (always start with 1 to 2 pounds) to avoid injury and ensure a positive result. While many people meet regularly with a certified trainer or exercise physiologist, you can also schedule two to four sessions to develop a routine that you can do by yourself. You might also look online for top-rated instructional DVDs to get you started.

**The Real You Twelve Easy Steps for Total Body Strength Training**

1. **Squats.** Stand with your back against the wall. Position your feet on the floor several feet away from the wall, hip width apart. Slowly slide your back down the wall, and squat down until the tops of your thighs are parallel to the floor and your knees are at a 90-degree angle. Hold for several seconds. Repeat 8 to 10 times.

2. **Leg Curls.** Start with legs together, feet flat on the floor. Hold on to a wall or the back of a chair for balance. Slowly lift your heel back as if you are going to kick your buttocks. Make sure that both knees stay parallel to each other. Slowly bring your heel back to the floor and repeat 8 to 10 times. Continue with other leg.

3. **Bent Over Row.** Kneel on a padded bench or a flat surface with your left knee, keeping your right leg on the floor. Support yourself with your left arm, while holding a weight (1 to 5 pounds) in your right hand. Lift the weight until your elbow is slightly higher than your back. Return the weight to the starting position. Repeat on the opposite side. Choose a weight allowing you to do 8 to 10 repetitions on each side.

4. **Modified Push-Up.** Start by kneeling on the floor. Place your hands at your sides, shoulder width apart, so you are on all fours. Keep knees together, slightly bent. Slowly lower your body so that your nose almost touches the ground and your elbows are close to a 90-degree angle. Try to keep your back straight. Push your body up, using your arms. Return to starting position and repeat 8 to 10 times.

5. **Side Lift.** Stand with your arms down at your sides, with a weight (1 to 5 pounds) in each hand. Lift arms up to side, but not past shoulder height. Choose weights allowing you to repeat 8 to 10 times.

6. **Shoulder Press.** Sit or stand with your back straight. Hold weights (1 to 5 pounds) in both hands. Bend your elbows, and hold the weights even at shoulder level; your palms should face forward. Press the weights overhead, keeping your elbows slightly bent. Return to starting position. Choose weights allowing you to repeat 8 to 10 times.

7. **Shoulder Shrugs.** Hang your shoulders down at your sides with weights (1 to 5 pounds) in hand. Pull your shoulders up toward your ears, and then release. Choose weights allowing you to repeat 8 to 10 times.

8. **Arm Curl.** Stand with your knees slightly bent and shoulder width apart. Keep your back straight and head up, holding weights (5 to 10 pounds) at your sides. Keep your palms facing outward, and slowly curl the weight up toward your shoulder. Don't curl your wrist! Lower the weight slowly to the starting position. Do not straighten your arm completely during extension, and keep your elbow slightly flexed. Choose weights allowing you to repeat 8 to 10 times. Repeat with your other arm.

9. **Tricep Extension.** Stand with knees slightly bent, one foot in front of the other. Place left hand on a bench or flat surface for balance. Keep your upper torso parallel to the bench. Take the weight (2 to 5 pounds) in your right hand. Bend your arm at the elbow and raise your elbow to shoulder height. Your elbow will be at a 90-degree angle with your palm facing your side. Press the weight back until your forearm is parallel to the floor, keeping your elbow in place. Slowly return to starting position. Repeat on other arm. Choose a weight allowing you to repeat 8 to 10 times on each arm.

10. **Pelvic Tilt.** Lie on your back with your back flat and knees bent. Place your arms at your sides. Lift your buttocks up and toward the ceiling, and hold for 5 to 10 seconds. Return to starting position. Repeat 8 to 10 times.

11. **Back Extension.** Lie on your stomach and extend both arms above your head. Tighten your buttocks as you raise one arm and

the opposite leg. Keep your arm straight and your toes pointed. Hold for 5 to 10 seconds, and repeat on opposite side. Repeat 8 to 10 times.

12. **Calf Raise.** Stand with your feet flat on the floor. Lift heels, keeping toes on the floor. Return to flat position. Repeat 8 to 10 times.

In addition to improving muscle mass, another benefit of strength training is that it reduces body fat. Higher muscle mass and lower body fat percentage often go hand in hand. Take a look at body fat percentages that are classified on a range of different physical types. While it's not necessary to be in the professional athlete range (much too low, and unrealistic for most of us!), there are some recommended cutoffs. *For women, aim for 25 percent, with a health goal of below 30 percent. For men, aim for 20 percent, with a health goal of less than 25 percent.* Wonder about this gender difference? It's caused by natural hormone patterns (women don't have the testosterone levels of men, among other things), resulting in normal but higher body fat percentages. Obtaining your body fat percentage is an important step toward understanding your body composition, or your fat-to-muscle ratio. This measurement complements your body mass index, a height-to-weight standardized ratio (see appendix A), to create a benchmark for your progress toward uncovering the Real You.

The most accurate measure of your body fat percentage is given with a professional test that determines the metabolic differences between muscle and fat. These include the newest technologies of whole body PET scanning or a Bod Pod (which uses air displacement). Older methods, which are very accurate, include underwater weighing, or using calipers. If these all sound like outer-space methods to you, a home scale with a body fat measure included can provide a reasonable—but not perfect—idea of your body fat. The home scale method can be useful for monitoring changes over time, and can at least give you an idea (accuracy varies with the quality of the scale) of where you're starting from. Body fat doesn't change as quickly as your weight, so a few times a year is sufficient.

**Body Fat Percentage**

| Classification | Women | Men |
|---|---|---|
| Essential Fat | 10%–12% | 2%–4% |
| Athletes | 14%–20% | 6%–13% |
| Fitness | 21%–24% | 14%–17% |
| Acceptable | 25%–31% | 18%–25% |
| Obese | Over 32% | Over 25% |

*Source*: American Council on Exercise

## Interval Training

Varying the intensity of your effort level at specific intervals during your activity can optimize calorie burning, as well as revitalize a boring activity. Interval training can be used for all activities—from walking to leaf raking, dancing, pushing the baby's stroller, and biking. The Real You Walking Plan, for example, demonstrates how to use interval training during a walk. It's easy!

There are two times when interval training is especially helpful:

1. When you're trying to raise your all-around intensity level, such as going from walking to jogging. Alternating a few minutes of jogging with your walking gets you started, and you can pace your progress by varying the walk/jog intervals.

2. When you're bored with your routine, but like the activity, you can play a mental game with yourself to speed up and slow down. For every ten minutes of a leisurely bike ride (or stationary bike), you might include three to five minutes of intense pedaling. It really does help to shake things up.

## Stretching/Flexibility

Stretching is always a good thing to do—and even counts as activity, whether you're stretching to warm up for another activity, or alone. The term "flexibility" refers to your ability to move your joint through its complete range of motion. Maintaining joint flexibility is essential to everyday activity, as well as providing an improved sense of well-being. A good stretch is like a big yawn—and can be an amazing stress reliever as well. It's best to get some experienced advice on how to stretch different body areas, both to learn the techniques and to make sure you are doing them properly, to avoid injury.

While you may choose to do specific stretching exercises for a particular body part, you might also like the all-around stretching offered in yoga, tai chi, Pilates, and other Eastern-origin activities. They enhance both greater flexibility and strength-training, when done regularly, and they also aid the mind-body connection (see page 114).

## Benefits of Stretching

- Improves and develops body awareness
- Increases joint flexibility
- Supports injury prevention
- Reduces muscle tension
- Increases relaxation
- Improves coordination by allowing greater ease of movement

## The Real You Total Body Stretch for Flexibility

1. **Neck Flexion.** Bend head forward slowly and hold for 10 to 20 seconds. Return to starting position.
2. **Neck Rotation.** Turn head slowly to look over left shoulder. Repeat on right side.
3. **Neck Lateral Rotation.** Tilt head toward shoulder. Repeat on other side.
4. **Shoulder Stretch.** Gently pull your elbow across your chest toward the opposite shoulder. Repeat on other side.
5. **Upper Back Stretch.** Place your hands shoulder-width apart on a ledge (countertop or back of chair). Let your upper body drop down as you keep your knees slightly bent. Keep your hips directly above your feet.
6. **Triceps Stretch.** Hold a towel in your right hand. Drape towel over your shoulder and down behind your back. Grasp bottom of towel

with your left hand. Climb your left hand up the towel, trying to grasp your right hand. Repeat on opposite side.

7. **Thigh Stretch.** Stand in front of a ledge (countertop or back of chair) to balance yourself. Keeping your left hand on the ledge and your left knee soft, bring your right foot up behind you. Hold the top of your right foot with your right hand and gently pull your heel toward your buttocks. Repeat on other side.

8. **Hamstring and Ankle Stretch.** Sit with one leg extended and heel on the floor. Pull your foot back, pointing your toes to the ceiling. Lean gently forward from the hips until you feel a stretch in the back of your thigh. Repeat on other side.

9. **Calf Stretch.** Stand close to the wall and put one foot in front of the other. Place hands on the wall for support. Bend your front knee and lean forward, keeping the back leg straight and keeping both heels on the floor. Repeat on the other side.

## Mind-Body Activity

Connecting our minds with our bodies takes a lot of effort. Does this connection have any real payoff when it comes to activity? Absolutely! While the calorie burn can be similar, there are a lot of value-added features when we are engaging our mind and body in the same activity. Stress relief is a clear benefit, which we can get with activities such as yoga, tai chi, and Pilates. These methods combine strength training and stretching, along with relaxation. A key feature of success and enjoyment with these activities comes down to your ability to focus your mind on the movement you're doing *at the moment.* This is a learning process, and it does not come easily. It can be done solo or in a group, appealing to a variety of activity temperaments.

The mind-body connection is nature's own biofeedback approach to stress management. These are the true double duty activities, both to burn calories and to reduce stress and contribute to a sense of emotional well-being. Look for an introductory class or a drop-in session in your community. Or rent a video or DVD to learn more about a particular activity.

Developing an activity strategy that integrates both mindfulness and physical demands can be a new experience, but it certainly is worth a try. At the very least, you've learned that about yourself and can select another type of activity more suited to your temperament. Best-case scenario: you've identified another tool for your activity toolbox. And when it comes to activity, the more tools you have, the better you are able to prevent boredom and to stay connected to your healthy lifestyle for the long term.

# 6

# Medical and Biological Tools
## Addressing Your Health Issues

Obesity is classified as a chronic illness. So why can't my doctor help me, you might ask? Why can't my doctor cure my weight problems like other sicknesses? The translation of this question often turns around to "my doctor can't (or won't) help me." Here's where an attitude adjustment can really help. Your doctor can help you with the medical issues related to your weight, and he or she is your number one tool in helping you identify biological factors that might be related to both weight gain and difficulty in losing weight. Plus, if you've got health problems related to your weight, medical management of these problems is a key component to long-term successful weight management.

I'm not talking about your doctor as a cheerleader, or as an adviser on the best low-calorie dessert. The medical tool is essential to any successful toolbox. If there is a biological reason related to your struggle, your doctor can help identify it. Ranging from medications that cause weight gain to metabolic reasons or active illness, your doctor (and other health-care professionals such as a physician assistant or nurse practitioner) can help identify and treat medical factors that can interfere with long-term weight loss.

If you're reading this now and can't remember the last time you went to your primary care doctor (or are not even sure if you have one), put down this book and make a call. Your weight-loss success may depend on it.

## How to Talk to Your Doctor about Your Weight

I'd like to provide some guidelines for how to talk to your doctor about your weight issues. Your doctor *does* care about your weight. While weight regulation is a combination of both biology and behavior, as you have been reading throughout this book, it's important to start a conversation with your doctor that is honest and open. You will need to acknowledge that you need help with *both* your biology and your lifestyle. The first step is a review of your own weight-related risk factors for health, considering each of the following categories:

Family history (genetics)

Present weight

Current lifestyle

Current medical illness

Smoking history

Stress management

Next, you'll want to review the following checklist of factors that might be sabotaging your ability to lose weight. Open your discussion with your doctor by reviewing these two lists together. There are tests to evaluate all of these biological saboteurs, and there are effective treatments to manage them. It's important to face the reality of your medical history, since even the best lifestyle effort can be overridden by biological factors. If you feel you're doing everything right and you're not losing weight, the medical tool is a must-do. Make it a point to have a yearly checkup with your primary care doctor. Some women double up with their care, using their annual visit with their gynecologist as their yearly general checkup, but I strongly urge you to also select and develop a relationship with a primary care doctor. Particularly when it comes to weight loss, two medical heads are better than one.

## Biological Barriers to Weight Loss

- Metabolic syndrome (including insulin resistance)
- Insulin-requiring diabetes
- Polycystic ovarian syndrome (PCOS)
- Thyroid gland problems
- Reproductive hormone issues
- Family history
- Medication-induced weight gain
- Mood disorders (depression)
- Sleep disturbances
- Your hunger and fullness thermostat—the brain

It's important to partner with your doctor to identify, and distinguish, the biological contributions to your weight gain from the behavioral ones. You must accept that you *cannot* control most of the biological barriers, but *do* have some control over the behavioral ones. That's why the BEAM Box works. You're not asking your doctor to work miracles (with magical thinking of some new medicine that must be coming soon), but to help you understand and manage your biology and medical needs, as an important—but not the only—part of your weight loss BEAM Box.

### Alison's Story
## I Can't Lose Weight No Matter What I Try

Alison, age twenty-five, felt she'd carried at least an extra 30 pounds since her teenage years. In the past three years, her weight continued to creep up, about another 15 pounds, despite her commitment to a consistently healthy lifestyle. She shared with me that she had never had regular periods but hadn't really thought much about it. She "basically was fine" except for her weight and had not seen her doctor since she graduated from college about two years earlier. She always felt that it was harder for her to lose weight, compared with other people. As we chatted about her weight, she said that she was somewhat alarmed at some body changes she had noticed over the past months, including excessive growth of facial hair and some velvety skin patches along her neck (called skin tags). She was so focused on her inability to lose weight that until we discussed how she was feeling, these biological issues did not come up.

Alison scheduled an appointment with her doctor and was diagnosed with polycystic ovarian syndrome. A hormonal disturbance that produces the symptoms she described, PCOS is often associated with weight gain and inability to lose weight, and is related to insulin resistance, which is another invisible symptom of the disorder. Insulin resistance strongly contributes to weight gain and inability to lose weight and is effectively treated with the prescription medication metformin. After a month on the medication, Alison found that her BEAM Box was working. She lost about 4 pounds a month, so by the end of five months she had lost about 20 pounds—half of her goal. She remains on metformin and is successfully managing her PCOS with her doctor. Her lifestyle plan is on track, and she is no longer discouraged by a lack of progress. With the correction of her insulin resistance, the same plan that wasn't working before is now providing consistent and steady weight loss.

An open and honest discussion with your doctor can help identify the best path—and tools—for your own weight-loss success. One size does not fit all, and a good starting point is for your doctor to arrange for lab tests to obtain a metabolic snapshot of your body. In addition to taking your height and weight to calculate your body mass index (see chart in appendix A), your doctor will want to make sure you have fasting baseline blood measures of these factors:

- Blood sugar (glucose)
- Fasting insulin
- Total cholesterol
- HDL (think "healthy" or "good" cholesterol)

- LDL (think "lousy" or "bad" cholesterol)
- Triglycerides
- Blood pressure
- Liver function tests

You should also know what your numbers mean:

| Blood | Healthy Range | Borderline | Health Risk |
|---|---|---|---|
| Total cholesterol | 200 or below | 200–240 | above 240 |
| LDL | 100 or less | 100–160 | above 160 |
| HDL | 60 or higher | 40–60 | below 40 |
| Blood pressure | 120/80 or less | 120/80–140/90 | above 140/90 |
| Triglycerides | below 150 | 150–200 | above 200 |

The good news is that even small changes in weight—just 5 to 10 percent off your starting weight—often improve some of these measures, depending on your starting weight. If you're at 200 pounds, even 10 pounds lost and kept off can often make a positive difference in your health.

# Sizing Yourself Up

While body weight and the related BMI are among the most popular ways to "size yourself up," there are a number of other ways to do so. Your doctor might use one or more of the following factors as another tool to estimate your risk and expand your medical plan.

Body weight

Body mass index (BMI)

Waist circumference

Body fat percentage

Lean body mass (muscle) percentage

It's the total picture that matters most. A larger waist, indicating more fat in your middle, called "visceral fat," is associated with major health risk.

So someone with an apple shape who is just overweight on the BMI chart but whose extra weight is centered in the middle with a larger waist could have more health risk than someone who is heavier in pounds. Generally, a waist size over 40 inches for men and more than 35 inches for women indicates increased risk.

I'm often asked about the connection between muscle mass and body weight. Since muscle weighs more than fat, it is possible for those with a high lean body mass (lots of muscle) and low body fat to have a BMI falling in the overweight range. Is that a bad thing? Typically, this unusual combination (overweight, but not overfat) is only seen among serious body builders and some professional athletes and doesn't apply to the vast majority of individuals. That's why most doctors will use at least two or more of these measurements to provide a comprehensive picture of how your weight affects your health. So it's not only the BMI that is important. In general, if you're overweight, it's likely from extra fat, not extra muscle, even if you lift weights. For body fat and muscle assessments not available in your doctor's office, you might consider asking for a referral.

## Janet's Story
### I'm Shaped Like an Apple

When she turned thirty, Janet made the decision to take charge of her health. She became a healthier eater, joined a walking group, and filled her BEAM Box with many effective strategies. While she was always trying to lose a few pounds, at this point in her life Janet was content with just not gaining weight, and remaining weight-stable. Then she quit her pack-a-day smoking habit—a major health triumph for her—but in the process gained 25 pounds. She was now concerned that her extra weight, concentrated in her abdomen, put her at an increased health risk: "I'm shaped like an apple, and I'm worried." She also struggled to just maintain her current weight and wondered if those extra pounds had somehow made it harder for her to lose weight. The only way to know was with some bloodwork, and I suggested a visit to her doctor to discuss the possible health implications of her apple shape. With a waist circumference of 36 inches, her abdominal fat could put her at increased risk for diabetes.

Her doctor determined that while Janet did not yet have a diagnosis of type 2 diabetes (her blood sugar was close to normal), she did have metabolic syndrome and was insulin resistant. This put her in the prediabetes category, with insulin levels that were too high and likely sabotaging even her best lifestyle effort. While her doctor was pleased with her efforts to lose weight, he added metformin, a medication to help lower insulin levels, which often results in a better rate of weight loss with a lifestyle effort. Janet was responsive to the medication and found that it made her effort to lose weight finally pay off. She began to see modest results—about 3 pounds a month. It took Janet about ten months to lose those 25 pounds. Much to her surprise, when she lost the extra weight, her doctor suggested discontinuing the medication. Janet no longer had metabolic syndrome—she got a clean bill of health.

# Talking to Your Doctor about the Power Tools: Prescription Medication and Surgery

When it comes to adding power tools to your BEAM Box, it's important for you to initiate the conversation about these additional tools with your doctor, not online with "Doctor Google." You are looking for additional options to make the lifestyle effort easier, but not to replace it. With the agreement that lifestyle must be the foundation of weight loss (you are not asking for miracles!), you'll be able to have a realistic chat with your doctor. There are pros and cons to both prescription medication and surgery, and these have to be discussed in practical terms for you: how they might affect other health factors, medications you already take, expectation of weight loss, plus financial considerations, among other topics.

The bottom line? When it comes to weight loss, you are a unique individual. Only a discussion with your doctor can help put your weight-related health risk into perspective and help you manage the biological factors contributing to your struggle with weight control. While some doctors are very engaged with the rest of the BEAM Box (eating, activity, behavior), most often you can expect your doctor to be supportive mainly of the medical tools and sometimes to help you with a reliable referral for building the other tools, including those power tools of prescription medication and surgery.

If you find that your doctor is less inclined to provide the kind of support you are seeking in building your own weight-loss BEAM Box, then it might be time to find another primary care doctor, or to network elsewhere for additional services. Ask friends and family members for their suggestions and referrals to help you in finding the right fit when it comes to your doctor.

### *Michael's Story*
## I've Got 100-plus Pounds to Lose

Michael came to see me with his wife, Nikki, his high school sweetheart. At thirty-six, Michael was a former high school football player who had bulked up on the coach's recommendation and had continued gaining weight in college and ever since. He needed to lose about 150 pounds. He was feeling scared and desperate, since he had developed high cholesterol in the past year. He hadn't returned to the doctor in more than a year, because he was afraid of more bad news and didn't want a lecture from his doctor about his climbing weight. Michael agreed that the combination of long work hours, business meals, and low physical activity had contributed to his steady weight gain, along with a strong family history of severe obesity (both of his parents are severely obese with health problems). He worked long days as an accountant and was trying to start his own small firm. He complained of constant fatigue. Michael and Nikki (age thirty-two) wanted to start a family, but they were concerned that Michael's severe obesity had to be addressed before this next big life step.

While Michael and I worked out a sustainable lifestyle plan for his BEAM Box, he agreed it was important for him to meet with his primary care doctor in order to identify any further medical issues relating to his weight that needed attention in order to support his overall health. Michael took both checklists and used this as the start of a conversation with his doctor. Much to his surprise, Michael's primary care doctor was happy to discuss weight loss with him and was pleased with his effort to lose weight. While Michael was disturbed that he now also had high blood pressure, for which he was prescribed medication, he was relieved that he had his doctor in the treatment loop.

Because of his chronic fatigue, Michael was also referred for a test for sleep apnea, an illness often associated with severe obesity, where the sleep cycle is severely interrupted multiple times a night, with a resulting poor night's sleep. He was diagnosed with sleep apnea and fitted with a CPAP (Continuous Positive Airway Pressure) machine to wear at night. With a regular good night's sleep, Michael was more energized and alert during the day and was able to sustain both his eating changes and his activity regimen. In his first six months, Michael lost 35 pounds.

Michael spent a lot of time thinking about his ability to sustain this effort with lifestyle alone and to continue to lose another 100 pounds. After discussion with Nikki, he felt he needed to add a power tool to sustain his effort and enthusiasm. With the support and referral of his primary care doctor, Michael was evaluated as a candidate for obesity surgery. His story continues in chapter 8.

---

# 7

# The Real You Plan
## BEAM Your Way to Success

**The twenty-one-day** Real You plan has two phases.

Phase one is the first seven days. Your first week is all about forming new habits. You'll start personalizing your lifestyle plan—what you eat, how you move, and how you manage daily stressors. A to-do list will get you jump-started. You'll be trying new tools or combining your old and trusted tools with some of the different tools that I've suggested.

For phase two, you'll take fourteen more days to sustain those new habits. Building on phase one, you'll be working for consistency and also fine-tuning your new habits—adjusting what you eat or when you eat, building on your daily activity, and testing out your various tools for the long haul.

If you haven't yet read and reviewed the four chapters describing the tool groups that will be the core foundation of your BEAM box, be sure to do that at the same time you are following the twenty-one-day plan. Unless you put together your individual effective BEAM Box with your personalized tools, you will not be setting yourself up for optimal success with this plan.

# TWENTY-ONE DAYS TO THE REAL YOU

## Phase 1: Creating Your Seven-Day Plan

It's in this first week that you'll start personalizing your lifestyle plan — what you eat, how you move, and how you manage daily stressors. The to-do list below offers you some of the basic tools to get started with. Remember that the tools listed are explained in more detail in chapters 3 through 6.

Create a daily lifestyle log, with pen and paper or small notebook, or with a spreadsheet (see "Lifestyle Logging" in chapter 4). It's important to keep track of your food intake, physical activity, sleep patterns, and daily life stressors, and to review your activities every day.

### THE SEVEN-DAY TO-DO LIST

**Behavior: Learn to manage your stress.**

- Practice deep breathing.
- Count to ten before responding to requests.
- Visualize yourself responding in a calm manner.
- Learn to say no.
- Recognize stress early to counteract it sooner.
- Take a two-minute walk.
- Drink a low-calorie warm beverage, such as herbal tea.

**Eating: Be an educated and mindful eater.**

- Keep your lifestyle log every day.
- Mix and match to satisfy your food preferences.
- Read food labels.
- Enjoy one or two snacks a day, to avoid getting over-hungry.
- Save a part of a meal (if you're already satisfied) for a snack.
- Use the Anytime Foods and Drinks to stay on track.
- Buy a calorie counter or use calorie information found online to validate your choices.
- Make sure to eat a morning meal within two hours of waking up.

**Activity: Make the effort to move more every day.**

- Wear your pedometer daily.
- Accumulate thirty minutes of walking daily.
- Aim for 5,000 steps daily in the first three days.
- Add 500 steps a day for a goal of 10,000 steps daily.
- Be consistent: include activity five to six days a week.
- Initiate activity daily, even if duration is shorter.
- Include one additional type of activity: strength, mind-body, cardio.

**Medical: Regulate your sleep patterns.**

- Avoid all sources of caffeine after 3 p.m. (such as soda, coffee, tea).
- Eat dinner at least two hours before bedtime.
- Consume an evening snack no later than one hour before bedtime.
- Limit or avoid liquids two hours before bedtime.
- Visit the bathroom immediately prior to getting in bed.
- Have a thirty- to sixty-minute relaxation ritual before bedtime (read, watch TV, drink herbal tea or skim milk).
- Aim for eight hours, but no less than seven hours, of sleep nightly.
- Keep your sleep/wake time cycle consistent.
- Take a power nap in the afternoon if needed.

## The Real You Seven-Day Meal Plan

The seven-day Real You meal plan provides a list of meals and snacks that you can mix, match, or divide in any way that suits you. The basic daily plan includes three meals and two snacks (five "eating episodes," as I like to call them), plus the Anytime Foods and Drinks. Your two snacks can be at any time of day, and if you want to eat even more often, then save part of your meal to eat as a snack. That's important because when you listen to your body for that Level 2 of fullness (where you feel content and satisfied, but you could eat more), it's time to stop, even when there's more food left in the meal.

It's a simple plan that provides structure without rigidity. You can follow it with as much or as little variety as you like. With this eating plan, you are *mindful* of calories and portions, but caloric precision is not necessary. If you focus on Level 2 of fullness, you will reconnect and relearn (or learn for the first time) that sense of satisfaction after eating without being stuffed.

Accept that your sense of contentment *will* change from day to day—sometimes you'll need another 100 calories or so to achieve Level 2 at a particular meal or from a snack. That's when you'll need to remind yourself that allowing for a little wiggle room with those extra calories means success in connecting with the Real You, rather than failure in going over some rigid calorie limit. This Real You meal plan is geared to help you jump-start your thinking about the kinds of foods and meals you prefer. Take a look at the variety of breakfast, lunch, and dinner suggestions and choose a basic eating pattern. You should feel free to choose any of the meals to eat at any time of day. It's important to get away from "eating by the clock" thinking. Chapter 4 has more discussion on food choices and how to mix and match, as well as how to keep restaurant eating consistent with your plan.

You'll notice that I've included some meal replacement shakes and bars as options for breakfast, lunch, or dinner. These are great when you're on the road or in a hurry and need a Plan B so you don't get derailed. They don't need refrigeration and are portable and convenient. You might consider them for one or even two meals a day, perhaps paired with a fresh fruit or vegetable.

Take a look at the Anytime Foods and Drinks. These are foods and drinks with few or no calories that you can eat freely to remain content and avoid deprivation.

Recipes marked with an asterisk can be found in the Real You Recipe File on page 211. While the recipe file is not an exhaustive one, it does represent many of my personal favorites. I've modified them to maintain great taste with far fewer calories and fat compared to traditional recipes. My family and friends find them delicious and satisfying. Plus, they're quick and easy to prepare.

**Seven Real You Breakfasts**

Easy Vegetable Frittata*

2 thin slices Canadian bacon (or prepackaged single-serve)

½ cup berries (fresh or frozen)

Coffee or tea (regular or decaf; skim/low-fat milk; low-calorie sweetener if desired)

PB and J Waffle*

8-ounce glass skim milk

Coffee or tea (regular or decaf; skim/low-fat milk; low-calorie sweetener if desired)

Quick and Tasty Egg Sandwich*

Coffee or tea (regular or decaf; skim/low-fat milk; low-calorie sweetener if desired)

Yogurt Parfait*

Coffee or tea (regular or decaf; skim/low-fat milk; low-calorie sweetener if desired)

High-protein ready-to-drink shake (Boost, Slim-Fast, and others under 300 calories per shake)

Medium apple

Coffee or tea (regular or decaf; skim/low-fat milk; low-calorie sweetener if desired)

1 pack Weight Control Instant Oatmeal (or any low-sugar brand)

1 small banana

1 cup skim milk

Coffee or tea (regular or decaf; skim/low-fat milk; low-calorie sweetener if desired)

1 cup Barbara's Puffins cinnamon cereal

½ cup fresh or frozen berries

1 cup skim milk

Coffee or tea (regular or decaf; skim/low-fat milk; low-calorie sweetener if desired)

Anytime Foods or Drinks (as desired)

## Seven Real You Lunches

Buffalo Chicken Fingers*

Carrot and celery sticks

100-calorie bag of chips (your choice)

1 tangerine

1 cup My Favorite Vegetable Soup*

Chicken Caesar Salad*

10 Melba Toast Rounds

1 medium fresh pear

Tuna-Spinach Wrap*

1 orange

Twist on a Cobb Salad*

15 Triscuit Thin Crisps

1 cup cut-up melon

Turkey sandwich (2 slices thin-sliced or low-calorie whole wheat bread; 3 ounces lean deli turkey; lettuce, tomato, and mustard)

1 cup tomato soup

100-calorie bag of pretzels or chips

½ cup red grapes

Calorie-controlled frozen pasta lunch entrée

Steam-in-the-bag broccoli or cauliflower

High-protein bar (South Beach, Balance, Zone, Kashi, Luna, and others under 300 calories per bar)

1 medium apple

Anytime Foods or Drinks (as desired)

**Seven Real You Dinners**

Marinated Grilled Flank Steak*

Roasted Green Beans*

¾ cup cooked whole wheat couscous

1 skinless barbecued chicken breast (or one quarter of a purchased rotisserie chicken, skin removed)

Cucumber and Onion Salad*

1 medium baked potato (white or sweet)

1 cup mixed berries (fresh or frozen)

Savory Shrimp Scampi*

½ cup whole wheat couscous

1 cup steamed green beans

1 cup steamed cauliflower

Crustless Peach Pie*

Hearty Meat Sauce*

2 ounces whole wheat or flax pasta

½ ounce shredded Parmesan cheese

Mixed raw greens

White Beans and Greens with Polenta*

One-Minute Baked Apple*

Large mixed green salad

2 tablespoons reduced-calorie dressing

Calorie-controlled single-serve frozen vegetable pizza

10 turkey pepperoni slices

Calorie-controlled dinner frozen meal (beef/chicken/fish main dish)
1 cup sugar snap peas (fresh or frozen)
1 cup steamed Brussels sprouts (fresh or frozen)
Anytime Foods or Drinks (as desired)

## Starter Menus for the Seven-Day Real You Plan

Remember, getting started is the hardest part. The Real You starter menus are designed to help guide you to an eating style that will work for you, but maybe not for someone else. There is no perfect way to eat in these first seven days. The goal is to both understand your preferences and give yourself permission to experiment with different kinds of food categories.

The starter menus provide variety in three key areas: (1) carbohydrate-focused (Carb); protein-focused (Prot); and on-the-go/easy prep (Easy). You don't need variety if you don't want it. You have seven different breakfasts, lunches, and dinners to choose from. You decide the structure and how much variety to include. If you like the same foods every day, fine. If you prefer more diversity, vary your meals to reflect that.

Within three days, you should get to a comfort level with the kinds of foods you enjoy and keep you satisfied. You can also barter and exchange with other foods within the same category (see chapter 4 for more on bartering). You'll be able to determine if you're an eater who is satisfied by eating more lean protein and fewer starchy carbohydrates, or if perhaps you seek greater volume from low-density foods containing lots of fiber, water, and air.

Experimenting with these menus will help you evaluate how often you need to adjust your foods. If your taste buds need a wake-up call more often, you'll want to change your foods more often to stay connected. Eating a high-protein breakfast of egg whites and Canadian bacon every day may work for you, even for weeks at a time, until it doesn't! Then you feel deprived and start looking for some starch. If that happens, switch to one of the carbohydrate-dense breakfasts. It's as easy as that. When it comes to food choice, change can be a very good thing. Learn to listen to and trust your body.

Some of these menus might look familiar to you, with a certain "comfort level" that works for you. If so, that's a great start. A major feature of developing your plan is to achieve structure, without rigidity, and get rid of the good-food-versus-bad-food mentality. As I've told you earlier, my mantra is that there are no bad foods, just bad portions. Keep this in mind when you're planning your own first seven days.

Recipes marked with an asterisk can be found in the Real You Recipe File on page 211.

## Day 1 (Prot)

*Breakfast:* Easy Vegetable Frittata*

*Lunch:* "Buffalo" Chicken Fingers*

*Dinner:* Marinated Grilled Flank Steak*

*Snack 1:* Laughing Cow light wedge with celery sticks

*Snack 2:* 6 ounces fat-free Greek-style yogurt

Anytime Foods and Drinks

## Day 2 (Carb)

*Breakfast:* PB and J Waffle*

*Lunch:* My Favorite Vegetable Soup,* Chicken Caesar Salad*

*Dinner:* Hearty Meat Sauce* with whole wheat pasta

*Snack 1:* ½ cup dry Kashi Good Friends Cereal

*Snack 2:* 100-calorie bag microwave popcorn

Anytime Foods and Drinks

## Day 3 (Easy)

*Breakfast:* High-protein, ready-to-drink shake; 1 apple

*Lunch:* Calorie-controlled frozen pasta lunch entrée

*Dinner:* Rotisserie chicken breast (purchased)

*Snack 1:* 1 large apple

*Snack 2:* 110-calorie Pria bar

Anytime Foods and Drinks

## Day 4 (Prot)

*Breakfast:* Yogurt Parfait*

*Lunch:* Tuna-Spinach Wrap*

*Dinner:* Savory Shrimp Scampi*

*Snack 1:* 2 fat-free Ball Park White Meat Turkey Hot Dogs

*Snack 2:* 1 low-fat provolone cheese stick; 2 thin slices deli turkey

Anytime Foods and Drinks

## Day 5 (Carb)

*Breakfast:* Low-sugar oatmeal (any brand) or Weight Control Oatmeal

*Lunch:* Tomato soup, turkey sandwich

*Dinner:* White Beans and Greens with Polenta*

*Snack 1:* Raw veggies and 100-calorie light ranch dip

*Snack 2:* 1 cup frozen cherries

Anytime Foods and Drinks

## Day 6 (Easy)

*Breakfast:* Barbara's Puffins cereal and skim milk

*Lunch:* Protein meal replacement bar; 1 apple

*Dinner:* Calorie-controlled frozen dinner, frozen vegetables

*Snack 1:* Low-fat ice cream novelty (80 to 120 calories)

*Snack 2:* Small skim-milk decaf latte

Anytime Foods and Drinks

## Day 7 (Mixed Options)

*Breakfast:* Quick and Tasty Egg Sandwich*

*Lunch:* Twist on a Cobb Salad*; Triscuit Thin Crisps; Fruit

*Dinner:* Calorie-controlled single-serving pizza and salad

*Snack 1:* 100-calorie pack of almonds or pistachio nuts (about 15 nuts)

*Snack 2:* 100-calorie bag Popchips

Anytime Foods and Drinks

# Phase 2: The Next Fourteen Days: Adjusting Your Plan to Sustain a Habit

The next fourteen days are when you should work on establishing consistency in your daily lifestyle, building on the base you created in the first seven days. Remember, it takes about three weeks to form a habit, so this two-week period is the best time to test out your selections for the long haul. Feel free to adjust your meals and snacks to keep yourself interested and engaged. Whether you are drawn to a higher-protein meal, need a change with a fiber-rich starch, or need more on-the-go choices, use this time to fine-tune your habits. Review the tools in your BEAM Box and modify them as needed to accommodate your changing needs if necessary.

## Phase 2 Meal Plans

Here are seven more days of Real You meals to add to your plan. I'm including more vegetarian meals for further variety. Or if you prefer to continue with more starter menus, then check out my suggestions for the next fourteen days in the next section. Again, feel free to mix and match according to your preferences. Once you've taken a look, see what changes you might like to incorporate. Or experiment outside of your "preference zone"—who knows, you might find a new favorite when you least expect it!

Remember, if you liked the first seven days, just stick with your new plan. By the end of twenty-one days, you should feel confident that you're able to sustain your present eating plan. If you're *not* feeling confident at this point, go back to Phase 1 and the first seven days of the plan. Review chapters 3 (Behavior), 4 (Eating), and 6 (Medical) to get some guidance on barriers that might be interfering with finding the Real You. With patience, personal insights, and sometimes professional help, you will succeed in developing a BEAM Box that works for you.

Recipes marked with an asterisk can be found in the Real You Recipe File on page 211.

## Seven More Real You Breakfasts

Fruit and Nut Oatmeal*

1 cup skim milk or soy milk

Coffee or tea (regular or decaf with skim or low-fat milk and low-calorie sweetener if desired)

Amy's Breakfast Burrito (in the freezer section)

½ cup fresh or frozen blueberries

Coffee or tea (regular or decaf with skim milk and low-calorie sweetener if desired)

Vitamuffin VitaTop (Cranbran or BluBran in the freezer section)

4 ounces nonfat sugar-free yogurt

Coffee or tea (regular or decaf with skim milk and low-calorie sweetener if desired)

Bagel 'n Lox*

1 cup melon, cubed

Coffee or tea (regular or decaf with skim milk and low-calorie sweetener if desired)

Carnation Sugar-Free Instant Breakfast drink (any flavor)
8 ounces skim milk

1 small banana

Coffee or tea (regular or decaf with skim milk and low-calorie sweetener if desired)

1 cup Special K Protein Plus cereal

6 ounces skim milk

½ cup fresh or frozen berries

Coffee or tea (regular or decaf with skim or low-fat milk and low-calorie sweetener if desired)

Tomato and Cheese Omelet*

3 slices tempeh bacon

½ cup grapes

Coffee or tea (regular or decaf with skim milk and low-calorie sweetener if desired)

Anytime Foods or Drinks (as desired)

## Seven More Real You Lunches

Tuna Tortilla*

1 medium fresh pear

Bumble Bee Ready-to-Eat Light Tuna Meal Kit

1 cup red grapes

Quick Chicken BLT Wrap*

½ cup raw mini carrots

100-calorie bag Popchips

Lean Pockets, any variety (available in the freezer section)

Celery and carrot sticks

8 ounces skim milk or skim soy milk

Bean Burrito*

1 tangerine

Lettuce Wraps*

½ cup frozen cherries

Taco Salad*

1 medium peach (or 1 cup frozen sliced peaches)

Anytime Foods or Drinks (as desired)

## Seven More Real You Dinners

Deluxe Veggie Burger* and Oven-Baked Garlic Fries*

Lettuce, tomato, red onions

1 medium apple

Baked Salmon and Asparagus*

1 small baked sweet potato

Mixed green salad with balsamic vinegar

Quick and Easy Stir Fry*

½ cup brown rice

½ cup no-sugar-added applesauce

Beef-Vegetable Kabobs*

½ cup whole wheat couscous

Easy Teriyaki Pork Tenderloin*

1 small baked white or sweet potato

1 cup steamed fresh or frozen broccoli

Turkey Cacciatore*

¾ cup cooked whole wheat penne (or other short-cut pasta)

1 cup steamed sugar snap peas

Hearty Mushroom Barley Soup*

1 slice light 100% whole wheat bread or small whole wheat pita bread

Mixed green salad

Anytime Foods or Drinks (as desired)

## Phase 2 Starter Menus

### Day 8 (Carb)

*Breakfast:* Fruit and Nut Oatmeal*

*Lunch:* Bean Burrito*

*Dinner:* Turkey Cacciatore*

*Snack 1:* 100-calorie pack Wheat Thins; Laughing Cow Light cheese wedge

*Snack 2:* 100-calorie microwave bag butter-flavor popcorn

Anytime Foods and Drinks

### Day 9 (Prot)

*Breakfast:* Tomato and Cheese Omelet*

*Lunch:* Lettuce Wraps*

*Dinner:* Beef-Vegetable Kabobs*

*Snack 1:* 6 ounces fat-free Greek-style yogurt with 1 tablespoon chopped walnuts

*Snack 2:* 100-calorie package whole raw almonds (or about 15 nuts)

Anytime Foods and Drinks

### Day 10 (Easy)

*Breakfast:* Carnation Sugar-Free Instant Breakfast drink

*Lunch:* Lean Pockets, any variety

*Dinner:* Quick and Easy Stir Fry*

*Snack 1:* Balance 100 Calorie bar

*Snack 2:* 1 medium banana

Anytime Foods and Drinks

### Day 11 (Carb)

*Breakfast:* Vitamuffin VitaTop

*Lunch:* Tuna Tortilla*

*Dinner:* Hearty Mushroom Barley Soup*

*Snack 1*: ¾ cup Barbara's Puffins peanut butter cereal

*Snack 2*: 100-calorie pack microwave kettle corn

Anytime Foods and Drinks

## Day 12 (Prot)

*Breakfast*: Special K Protein Plus cereal

*Lunch*: Taco Salad*

*Dinner*: Baked Salmon and Asparagus*

*Snack 1*: Fat-free hot dog and 1 low-fat provolone stick

*Snack 2*: 3 slices white meat turkey (prepackaged or deli-counter)

Anytime Foods and Drinks

## Day 13 (Easy)

*Breakfast*: Amy's Breakfast Burrito

*Lunch*: Bumble Bee Ready-to-Eat Light Tuna Meal Kit

*Dinner*: Easy Teriyaki Pork Tenderloin*

*Snack 1*: 1 medium fresh apple

*Snack 2*: 90-calorie rice pudding cup

Anytime Foods and Drinks

## Day 14 (Mixed)

*Breakfast*: Bagel 'n Lox*

*Lunch*: Quick Chicken BLT Wrap*

*Dinner*: Deluxe Veggie Burger* and Oven-Baked Garlic Fries*

*Snack 1*: ½ cup low-fat ice cream, frozen yogurt, or single-serve ice cream novelty (70 to 120 calories)

*Snack 2*: ½ cup grapes and 1 low-fat Bonbel mini cheese

Anytime Foods and Drinks

Okay, now you've been working on the Real You eating plan for two weeks. You should be on your way to some solid habits you can sustain over the long term. During this third week, mix and match some of your favorite meals using meal-to-meal change, and daily or weekly variations. Here's another seven days of menus, to complete your first twenty-one days. If you don't quite feel that your habits are completely formed, keep going for another seven days and adjust your eating pattern. Everyone is different. While it *does* take about three weeks to form a new habit, the key word here is "about." You might need four weeks, or even five, until you hit your meal plan stride and truly find the real you.

### Day 15 (Prot)

*Breakfast:* Easy Vegetable Frittata*

*Lunch:* Buffalo Chicken Fingers*

*Dinner:* Marinated Grilled Flank Steak*

*Snack 1:* Laughing Cow Light wedge with celery sticks

*Snack 2:* 6 ounces fat-free Greek-style yogurt

Anytime Foods and Drinks

### Day 16 (Easy)

*Breakfast:* High-protein, ready-to-drink shake; 1 apple

*Lunch:* Calorie-controlled frozen pasta lunch entrée

*Dinner:* Rotisserie chicken breast (purchased)

*Snack 1:* 100-calorie package raw almonds (about 15 nuts)

*Snack 2:* 100-calorie bag microwave popcorn

Anytime Foods and Drinks

### Day 17 (Carb)

*Breakfast:* PB and J Waffle*

*Lunch:* My Favorite Vegetable Soup,* Chicken Caesar Salad

*Dinner:* Hearty Meat Sauce* with whole wheat pasta

*Snack 1:* ½ cup dry Quaker Crunchy Corn Bran cereal

*Snack 2:* 100-calorie bag microwave popcorn

Anytime Foods and Drinks

## Day 18 (Mixed)

*Breakfast:* Bagel 'n Lox

*Lunch:* Quick Chicken BLT Wrap*

*Dinner:* Deluxe Veggie Burger* and Oven-Baked Garlic Fries*

*Snack 1:* ½ cup low-fat ice cream, frozen yogurt, or single-serve ice cream novelty (70 to 120 calories)

*Snack 2:* ½ cup grapes and 1 low-fat Bonbel mini cheese

Anytime Foods and Drinks

## Day 19 (Prot)

*Breakfast:* Yogurt Parfait*

*Lunch:* Tuna-Spinach Wrap*

*Dinner:* Savory Shrimp Scampi*

*Snack 1:* 2 Fat-Free Ball Park White Meat Turkey Hot Dogs

*Snack 2:* 1 low-fat provolone cheese stick; 2 thin slices deli turkey

Anytime Foods and Drinks

## Day 20 (Carb)

*Breakfast:* Low-Sugar or Weight Control Oatmeal

*Lunch:* Tomato soup, turkey sandwich

*Dinner:* White Beans and Greens with Polenta*

*Snack 1:* Raw veggies and 100-calorie light ranch dip

*Snack 2:* 1 cup frozen cherries

Anytime Foods and Drinks

## Day 21 (Easy)

*Breakfast:* Amy's Breakfast Burrito

*Lunch:* Packaged Tuna Meal Kit

*Dinner:* Easy Teriyaki Pork Tenderloin*

*Snack 1:* 1 medium fresh apple

*Snack 2:* 90-calorie rice pudding cup

Anytime Foods and Drinks

# The Real You Starter Snack List

I'm often asked what counts as a snack. My bottom line with snacking is that it's a mini eating episode, ranging from 50 to 150 calories, to help you maintain a level of *contentment* but not feel stuffed. It's what I call the Level 2 of fullness. It's sometimes hard to separate "head" hunger from "physical" hunger, which is why snacking is such a challenge for most of us. It's important to understand that we really don't need to refuel all day to keep our energy up and our blood sugar stable.

You might find that three structured meals each day work best for you, with some of the Anytime Foods and Drinks sufficiently satisfying. If you're looking for a snack, it's best to plan for the longest interval between your three main meals. For most people, a late-afternoon snack is a must-have, to bridge the time between lunch and dinner. Many people also seek a second snack, either between breakfast and lunch or between dinner and bedtime. The trick (which is no trick) is to choose the right kind of snack to satisfy both your energy needs and your particular food preferences. When it comes to snacking, the fullness factor we seek can be achieved with a variety of foods.

I'm a big fan of single-serving packaging. While most products are available in 100-calorie serving sizes, many companies now provide 50- to 60-calorie servings of some of your favorites, from yogurt to pretzels to low-fat cheeses. Even though it can be pricier, it gives you the immense satisfaction of eating to the bottom of the bag. It's a way of giving yourself permission to eat the whole thing. (You can create the same effect more economically by dividing up a large bag or box into individual servings in small plastic bags.) Don't minimize this important mental satisfaction of eating.

Of course, I'm also a big fan of using fresh fruits and vegetables as a snack, and I hope you are, too. It's a good idea, I think, to have a selection of go-to snacks that provide a different (not necessarily better) kind of taste and texture. Remember, you're looking for about 100 calories, to provide both mental and biological satisfaction.

**My Favorite Carbohydrate Snacks**

100-calorie pack microwave popcorn

100-calorie pack Popchips

½ 100-calorie English muffin with thin slice of low-fat cheese

Flatouts Wrap (multigrain with flax)

100% whole wheat matzoh sheet

Pria 110 bar

100-calorie pack Wheat Thins

100-calorie pack of dried fruits (cranberries, raisins, or apricots)

Balance 100 bar

1 cup Kashi Good Friends Cereal

1 cup Fiber One Raisin Bran Flakes

1 cup Barbara's Puffins cereal (any variety)

1 cup Quaker Crunchy Corn Bran cereal

1 medium sliced apple dipped in cinnamon

Small banana, spread with 1 teaspoon of peanut butter

100- to 150-calorie single-serving frozen ice cream treat

1 low-fat string cheese; 6 Triscuit Thin Crisps

I cup frozen cherries or blueberries (right from the freezer)

Clif Kid Twisted Fruit Rope

**My Favorite Protein Snacks**

Light string cheese

Laughing Cow Light low-fat Babybel cheese

4 ounces skim milk and ¾ cup Special K Protein Plus cereal

4 ounces low-fat cottage cheese

4 ounces fat-free, sugar-free yogurt

Single-serve fat-free Greek-style yogurt

Fat-free beef hot dog (Hebrew National, Ball Park)

Fat-free White Meat Turkey Frank (Ball Park)

3 thin slices low-salt deli turkey or ham

Small skim-milk decaf latte

100-calorie pack of almonds

Single-serve pack (120 calories) of pistachio nuts in shells

Soy burger (Boca or other brands)

## The Real You Anytime Foods and Drinks

It's important to be able to keep your mouth busy without consuming a lot of extra calories. That hand-to-mouth connection is a real challenge to break for most of us (more on that in chapter 3). It's great to have some fallbacks for when you want to satisfy an oral urge but not take in a lot of calories. This is the best way to avoid that feeling of deprivation leading to overeating. Here are some of my favorites. Feel free to rely on one or more of these anytime during the day or evening. You can also add your own favorites.

Bottled or tap water (with lemon, lime, or cucumber slices)

Seltzer/club soda

Herbal tea

Decaf coffee

Diet soda (limit to 24 ounces daily)

"Light" juice (10 to 20 calories per 8 ounces; limit to 20 ounces daily)

Sugar-free gelatin

Sugar-free ice pops

Sugarless gum (cinnamon)

Clear broth (chicken, beef, or vegetable)

My Favorite Vegetable Soup*

Dill pickle

Raw greens (cabbage, romaine, escarole, butter lettuce, red-leaf lettuce, green-leaf lettuce, baby greens)

Raw vegetables

All plain frozen bagged vegetables (except peas, corn, and potatoes)

## Managing Food Cravings

Whether it's biology or behavior, there are certain foods we just get a yearning for. So, what to do? Ignoring our cravings leads to deprivation, overeating, and guilt. Disconnecting and "giving in" leads to overeating and guilt. I'd like to suggest that you become a smarter eater when it comes to food cravings. Your goal is to satisfy, without triggering overeating. That's where the challenge is, and that's where a snack differs from a food that triggers craving: you want to identify a small amount of the desired food to *satisfy*. It's particularly important to keep about 100 calories in mind for that one-two punch of both biological and mental satisfaction. Check out chapter 4's section on trigger foods for more ideas.

Avoiding deprivation is essential for short- and long-term success, because the more you say no, the more deprived you feel, and you enter that downward spiral of losing control, overeating, feeling guilty, and giving up. In managing your food cravings, you gain confidence in being able to understand and control them. Here are some examples of simple and practical solutions to managing the four most common categories of food cravings.

**Salty/Crunchy**

Any 100-calorie bag of chips (Popchips, popcorn, reduced-fat regular potato chips, baked chips, Wow chips)

Single-serve bag of mini rice cakes (90 to 100 calories)

Large, crunchy dill pickle

15 Triscuit Thin Crisps

Raw celery and carrots with 2 tablespoons fat-free ranch dressing

1 whole bag salad greens (eaten right from the bag)

## Chocolate

4 dark or milk chocolate Hershey kisses

4 mini Tootsie Rolls

2 mini squares of Lindt 70% chocolate

100-calorie pack M&M's (or other "fun size" candy bar)

60-calorie Hershey's Special Dark chocolate sticks

100-calorie pack Nabisco Oreo Thin Crisps

100-calorie pack Hostess mini-chocolate cupcakes

4 chocolate-covered strawberries

25-calorie hot chocolate (Nestlé, Swiss Miss, or other)

Single-stick Fudgesicle (regular, not sugar-free or fat-free)

## Sweet Tooth

1 cup frozen cherries

100-calorie bag Craisins

100-calorie bag raisins

Freeze-dried fruits

4 chocolate-dipped strawberries

Single-serve bags of Sunkist apricots

Individually wrapped Sunkist prunes

2 Dum Dum lollipops

100-calorie pack gummy bears

Individually wrapped fruit-flavored Life Savers

100-calorie pack of Swedish fish

Single-wrapped Twizzler

Individually wrapped Creme Savers candy

Dentyne Fire cinnamon-flavored sugar-free gum

Fun-size box of Hot Tamales candy

Clif Kid Twisted Fruit Rope

### Fat Tooth (Smooth and Creamy)

Single-serve Kozy Shack sugar-free rice pudding

Jell-O sugar-free pudding—all varieties (60 calories)

Single-serve Greek-style 0% fat plain yogurt

Single-serve Skyrus yogurt—plain, vanilla, or fruit flavor

Weight Watchers 90-calorie Latte Bar

Skinny Cow ice cream cup or other novelty

Edy's single-serve cup of double-churned low-fat ice cream

Small (8–10 ounce) skim milk latte

Small (½ cup) Dairy Queen or Tasti D-lite soft-serve dish

### Three Steps to Satisfying Food Cravings

1. Think *before* you choose a food.
2. Pick a single-serving size so you can eat the whole thing.
3. Limit your portion to 150 calories or less.

# THE REAL YOU PANTRY SURVIVAL GUIDE

## Creating a Healthy Kitchen

The best thing about home cooking is that you definitely know what's in your food. You can't be fooled by hidden fats, and you've got better control over your serving sizes. Here are some of my favorite ways to save fat and calories when you're cooking at home.

## Low-Fat Cooking Methods

- Bake.
- Steam.
- Broil.
- Microwave.
- Grill.
- Roast poultry without the skin.
- Stir-fry or sauté using a nonstick pan coated with cooking spray.
- Use high-quality flavorful oil. (Limit 1 tablespoon per person.)

## Low-Fat, Low-Calorie Flavor-Boosters

- Dried and fresh herbs: basil, oregano, cilantro, parsley, thyme, rosemary
- Spices: cinnamon, nutmeg, paprika, pepper, lemon pepper, cardamom
- Mustard
- Ketchup
- Salsa
- Low-sodium soy sauce
- Reduced-fat or fat-free sour cream
- Reduced-fat or fat-free salad dressing
- Reduced-fat or fat-free mayonnaise
- Dijonnaise
- Lemon juice and lime juice
- Vinegar
- Horseradish
- Fresh and dried ginger
- Red pepper flakes
- Finely grated Parmesan or Romano cheese
- Sodium-free herb and pepper blends

## More Low-Fat Cooking Tips

- When broiling or roasting, elevate meat on a cooking rack so natural fat drips away.

- Look for "loin" and "round" when shopping for leanest cuts of beef and pork.
- Thin-sliced meat/poultry cooks quicker, with very little added fat.
- Use herb and spice rubs for calorie-free flavor.
- Use an oil cooking spray.
- Marinate in juices, flavored vinegars, and low-fat dressings instead of oil-based marinades.
- Trim away any visible fat on foods before cooking.

### Some Calorie-Saving Kitchen Tools

- Roasting rack that allows fat to drip away from meat
- Strainer to drain fatty and salty liquids
- Grater for small amounts of flavorful additions such as hard cheese or chocolate
- Fat-separating measuring cup to separate fat from flavorful pan juices
- Food scale to measure raw and cooked portion sizes (occasional use)
- Apple corer/slicer to effortlessly cut an apple for easy eating
- Infant/baby spoons or chopsticks for tasting while cooking
- Steamer basket for steaming vegetables, fish, and/or chicken
- Nonstick skillets and cookware for oil-free or limited-oil cooking
- Oil-spray can for use with high-quality, high-flavor oils

# Supermarket Shopping Tips

A few basic ground rules will go a long way toward supporting your BEAM Box. Most of us don't realize how important smart shopping in the market can be to a successful lifestyle plan. In fact, your shopping strategy starts *before* you even set foot in the grocery store.

### Before You Go to the Supermarket

- **Plan your meals for the week.** Invest some time in this, to save both money and calories. With planning, you buy only what you need and avoid impulsive purchases of high-calorie foods. If it's not around, you won't eat it. You can always leave a little wiggle room for adapting your meals to take advantage of in-store specials on fresh foods.

- **Make a list and shop from it.** When your meals are planned, you can make a complete list of items you'll need for the week. Stick to your list, and you'll limit impulse buying, a major problem for all of us.
- **Eat before you shop.** Have a snack before shopping, or go after a meal, to make sure you stick to your list. When you're hungry, it's hard to resist overbuying, even when you have a list. When you're content, you'll be much less likely to make impulsive buys for high-calorie foods. Believe me, it works.
- **Allow enough time to shop leisurely.** If you're in a hurry and multitasking, grocery shopping is just one more thing to add to a hectic day, making you more likely to grab and go and make less healthful choices. Give yourself enough time to read labels and comparison shop for calories, nutrient density, and cost. Take along only those family members who are willing to support your healthful purchases.
- **Use coupons to experiment with new foods.** While many popular coupons are for high-calorie snacks and packaged products, you'll find a variety of coupons for different kinds of high-fiber cereals, yogurts, calorie-controlled frozen foods, and other new offerings in these food categories. Buying these products can sometimes be a pricey experiment if you're not sure if you'll like them, so using a coupon is a good way to be an adventurous eater. Throw out any coupons for high-calorie snacks. If you take them to the store, you might be tempted to use them. Out of sight, out of mind.

## At the Market

- **Shop the perimeter of the store first.** The outside of the store is where all the fresh selections are. Many stores begin with the produce section, followed by meat/poultry/seafoods, the deli counter, and the dairy and egg cases. There are some variations to this pattern (dairy and eggs first and produce last), but you'll always find the fresh products around the outside of the store. Fill two-thirds of your cart with these items before you go down the middle aisles. That's where you'll find all of the boxed, canned, jarred, and frozen items. Shop those aisles *after* you've made the outer circuit. You simply won't have room for a lot of products with added calories, fat, and salt.

- **Chew some sugarless gum.** Or if you're not a gum-chewer, try a mint. Keeping your mouth busy will also help you avoid the variety of free samples of products offered throughout the store. It's often a meal in itself, by the time you've made it up and down all the aisles.
- **Use a calculator (or your phone or PDA).** When you need to calculate serving size and number of servings per package, it can be useful to have something on hand to do it quickly and easily. Plus, if you want less than the serving size stated on the package, you can quickly figure it out.
- **Get family members to cooperate.** It's best if you can shop alone, to read labels and think about your choices. If you've got your children or your partner along, make sure they are goal-oriented. No whining for junk that is not on the list. To avoid this, make sure that *before* you go shopping you put a treat food or two on the list to satisfy them. That's only fair, and it's also necessary for balanced eating! Remember the mantra of the Real You plan: "There are no bad foods, just bad portions."

Okay, let's take the real you shopping. Get your cart and take a virtual supermarket tour along with me. We'll go aisle by aisle through the grocery store. By developing and practicing your shopping skills, you'll be able to save time, calories, and money.

## Produce

Your three key words in the produce section are: (1) color, (2) variety, and (3) seasonal. Fresh and in-season fruits and vegetables are your top choices and most economical selections. You'll pay more for the convenience of cut-up and bagged selections or out-of-season produce, so think about these as you shop. A sharp knife and a cutting board may be a better way to go. Plus, think of the frozen aisle for out-of-season fruits; you get the same nutrition with better flavor and lower cost.

When shopping for produce, it is important to consider color, since phytochemicals, those plant nutrients responsible for color, provide value-added health benefits. Each color in the healthy produce rainbow supplies a different set of nutrients. While the jury is still out on the specifics of exactly *how* these power nutrients promote good health, a variety of research studies show a strong link between consumption and a positive health benefit. While most fruits and vegetables are both fiber- and water-rich (two immediate health pluses), here's a list of the individual colors and the various nutrients they indicate. All of these phytochemicals (plant nutrients) are potent antioxidants, which positively influence a variety of metabolic pathways in our bodies.

## Red

> *Color-producing power nutrient:* lycopene
>
> *What it does:* linked to heart health, cancer prevention
>
> *Where it's found:* tomatoes, watermelon, pink grapefruit

## Blue/Purple/Dark Red-Purple

> *Color-producing power nutrients:* anthocyanins, flavanols
>
> *What they do:* linked to heart and brain health, cancer prevention
>
> *Where they're found:* blueberries, blackberries, eggplant, currants, grapes, red cabbage, radicchio, red onions, raisins, plums, red pears, red apples

## Yellow-Orange

> *Color-producing power nutrient:* beta-carotene
>
> *What it does:* linked to heart health, cancer prevention
>
> *Where it's found:* sweet potatoes, pumpkin, oranges, tangerines, apricots, cantaloupe, carrots, mangoes, peaches, papaya

## Green

> *Color-producing power nutrients:* lutein, zeaxanthin
>
> *What they do:* linked to support of eye health

*Where they're found:* medium and dark green leafy vegetables, dark green salad greens, broccoli, Brussels sprouts, green beans, honeydew melon, kiwi, green peppers, asparagus

## White

*Color-producing power nutrient:* allium

*What it does:* linked to heart health and cancer prevention

*Where it's found:* onions, leeks, garlic, mushrooms, scallions

## Produce Checklist

*Fruits:* apples, apricots, bananas, blueberries, cantaloupe, cherries, clementines, cranberries, grapefruit, grapes, honeydew, kiwis, lemons, limes, mango, oranges, papaya, peaches, pears, pineapple, plums, raspberries, starfruit, strawberries, tangerines, watermelon.

*Vegetables:* artichokes, asparagus, bagged salad greens, beets, broccoli, Brussels sprouts, butternut squash, cabbage (green or red), carrots, cauliflower, celery, chili peppers, corn, cucumber, fennel, garlic, green beans, green leafy vegetables (collards, kale, Swiss chard), leeks, mushrooms, okra, onions, parsnips, peas, potatoes (white or sweet), salad greens (medium and dark green), spinach, squash, tomatoes, zucchini.

# Deli/Prepared Foods

Here's a section that will save you time, providing multiple items for a meal or a quick snack. Personalize your selections by having your cold cuts sliced fresh, extra-thin, with wax paper in between to keep the slices from sticking together. Ask questions, and choose carefully to avoid hidden calories and fat.

## Deli Checklist

Reduced-fat cheese

Turkey

Lean ham

Lean beef (such as eye of round)

Turkey pastrami

Chicken (all varieties: barbecued, smoked, roasted; ask for low-salt if available)

Rotisserie chicken or turkey (serve with skin removed)

## Fresh Meats/Poultry/Fish

There's a lot of choice here, which can be a calorie-savings or a disaster, unless you read the packaging. If you're shopping at the fresh butcher counter, make sure to add your special requests, like trimming extra visible fat, preportioning chicken breasts into 6-ounce pieces, or grinding a fresh turkey breast (for use as a tasty red-meat burger alternative).

### Meat/Poultry/Fish Checklist

*Red Meat:* ground beef (at least 90 percent lean; it's available as high as 96 percent lean), top round, top sirloin, flank steak, beef roast (eye of round), beef tenderloin, lamb roast leg, veal roast, veal scallopini cutlets (thin sliced).

*Poultry:* chicken breasts, thin-sliced chicken cutlets, chicken breast tenders, white turkey breast (whole or cutlets).

*Fish:* all varieties, avoiding breaded or stuffed options.

*Related Products:* 100 percent white-meat turkey hot dogs, low-fat beef hot dogs, fat-free hot dogs, low-fat kielbasa, Canadian bacon, soy hot dogs.

## Dairy

The dairy aisle is an easy section to navigate. Stick with low-fat and non-fat dairy products of all types. Read the labels carefully, as there is often a small calorie difference between a reduced-fat and a nonfat product. If you're new to low-fat dairy, try switching from full-fat to low-fat (not fat-free) for a few weeks. A change to fat-free will be too much of a shock to your taste buds. Even if you remain a reduced-fat dairy user, you will still get a significant savings of calories and fat.

### Dairy Checklist

Reduced-fat or fat-free milk, yogurt, cheese, and puddings; sugar-free fruited yogurts; reduced-fat or fat-free soy milk, yogurt, and cheeses; reduced-fat coffee creamer (or simply substitute 2 percent for whole milk); reduced-fat or fat-free calcium-fortified cottage cheese; reduced-fat or fat-free cream cheese; reduced-fat cheese sticks; reduced-fat Laughing Cow wedges or individual wax-wrapped pieces; reduced fat or fat-free sour cream; low-fat margarine; whipped butter; low-calorie butter spray.

*Related Products*: large eggs (brown or white), reduced-cholesterol eggs (optional), prepackaged egg substitute, prepackaged egg whites, low-fat firm tofu, hummus.

## Bread

I love the variety of fiber-rich, portion-controlled breads, rolls, bagels, and English muffins now available in the bread aisle. Don't just grab and go, since many of these products look the same but have widely different calorie and fiber content. Be a label reader in this aisle and you'll be sure to choose wisely. Remember, a dark bread can simply have some added coloring, which doesn't mean it's a whole grain. It's easy to be fooled when the label says "wheat." The key words here are "100% whole wheat." Look for serving size, calories per serving, and fiber content for optimal selections.

### Bread Checklist

100% whole wheat thin-sliced bread and sandwich buns, light (reduced-calorie) 100% whole wheat bread, mini pita breads (whole wheat or white), thin-sliced rye bread, thin-sliced seven-grain bread, Thomas's 100-calorie bagels, Weight Watchers bagels and English muffins, Thomas's 100-calorie 100% whole wheat English muffins, light (reduced-calorie) hamburger and hot dog buns, 100-calorie Arnold sandwich thins, Flatout wraps (multigrain with flax), small (6-inch) whole wheat fresh tortillas

## Beverages

When you remember that clear doesn't mean calorie-free, you're already off to a good start. As a general rule, stick with water or calorie-free seltzer. These should be your foundation. Or stick with your home tap water. Nervous about the quality? Attach a filter to your tap, or use a filter pitcher for your fridge. Don't even think about buying regular soda, even in smaller serving sizes. Diet sodas are a good option to supplement, but not replace, fluid intake from water on occasion. Even for sports activities, water is the best choice for most activities that last under an hour; a better choice is a lower-calorie and lower-sugar sports beverage, such as Propel, Powerade Zero, and G2 (Gatorade).

**Beverage Checklist**

Bottled water (all brands), seltzer, diet soda (all brands), Propel, G2, Powerade Zero.

## Canned Foods

Canned foods have a long shelf life, are economical, and can fill in when pricey fresh produce is out of season. You can purchase fruits canned in their own juice or in water, and low-salt canned vegetables and soups. The most economical canned fruits often have sugary syrups, and the vegetables and soups are often salt-laden. You can save money by buying these products and "cleaning" them up by rinsing them in a strainer under running water.

**Canned Foods Checklist**

Fruits (packed in their own juice or water), reduced-calorie juices (later you can mix half and half with water), sugar-free juices, low-sodium tomato and V8 juice, applesauce (no sugar added), low-sodium canned and boxed soups (no cream-based soups), light tuna packed in water (can or pouch), white meat chicken, pink or red salmon, canned beans (black, kidney, pinto, cannellini), vegetarian baked beans, vegetarian chili, vegetables (low-salt if available).

## Pasta/Rice/Grains

There are boxes and packaged items galore in this aisle. Two basics to look for here are: (1) whole grains and (2) simple ingredients. The "meal in a box" is to be avoided. Read the label to find out if your choice is a *whole grain* product. A big clue is the fiber content: a whole grain will provide at least 3 to 4 grams of fiber per serving, and up to 7 or 8 grams. As with breads, color doesn't indicate high nutrient content. A green "spinach" pasta is not a vegetable! In fact, the spinach content is virtually zero.

### Pasta/Rice/Grains Checklist

Brown rice (slow-cook or instant), quinoa, cracked wheat, bulgur, couscous, whole wheat pasta, flax pasta, kasha (buckwheat groats), wild rice, all whole grain mixtures without sauce.

## Meal and Snack Bars/Hot and Cold Cereals

The choices here vary from whole grain, nutrient-dense, calorie-controlled products to candy bars masquerading as health foods. Look beyond the promotional language on the package to find out what's inside. A picture of wheat on the package, or a label screaming "contains whole grains" is not convincing. Watch out for products like granola that sound natural but are loaded with extra calories and fat, often with limited nutrient density. When it comes to cereal products, you've really got to read below the headlines! Portion control is essential, as many cereals are loaded with fiber and whole grain but are calorie-dense. If you're using the cereal as a snack, you don't need to consume the package serving size, which usually is one cup; try a half-cup serving for a major calorie savings (usually around 100 calories).

When shopping for cereals, look for high-fiber products such as Fiber One cereal, Barbara's Puffins, Special K Protein Plus, All-Bran and

Bran Buds, Kashi Good Friends and other Kashi products. Oat products include Cheerios and unflavored oatmeal (large package or single-serve), or low-calorie flavored weight-control oatmeal in banana nut, cinnamon, or maple walnut flavors (single-serve).

Bars for meal replacement should have at least 4 grams of fiber, 8 grams of protein, and around 200 calories. Snack bars should have about half that number of calories. Easy choices are those made by South Beach, which sells both meal replacement bars (around 200 calories) and snack bars (around 100 calories). Cheerios makes cereal bars with added calcium, to approximate an on-the-go version of cereal and milk. Fiber One snack bars can give a big boost to your fiber intake. Read the labels carefully. Many granola and snack bars have health-promoting packaging but very little nutritional content when you read the fine print.

## Coffee/Tea/Hot Chocolate/Drink Mixes

While many people focus on the caffeine in this aisle, it's important to make sure you're buying a sugar-free, low-calorie item, whether it's a brewed or an instant product.

### Coffee/Tea/Hot Chocolate/Drink Mix Checklist

All brewed and instant coffees (caffeinated or decaf), all brewed and instant regular or herbal (floral) teas, Nestlé fat-free 25-calorie hot chocolate, Swiss Miss 50-calorie hot chocolate with calcium, sugar-free coffee beverages (such as cappuccino), single-serve powdered sachets of Crystal Light, 4C lemonade, flavored ice tea (sugar-free), Propel, or other similar low-calorie drink packets.

## Chips/Cookies/Crackers

If there's one aisle where prepackaged 100-calorie foods are your friend, it's the chips and cookies aisle. If you don't want the expense of prepackaged portion control, stop in the plastic wrap aisle for some snack-size food storage bags to make your own 100-calorie (or even 50-calorie) snack packs. Avoid fat-free cookies—the calories are virtually the same as in the real thing (and sometimes more!). When it comes to fat, pay attention in crackers. Here's where you'll want to look at fat content first, to avoid a lot of invisible calories. And you always want to steer clear of trans fats.

### Chips/Cookies/Crackers Checklist

All trans-fat-free chips, cookies, and crackers; fiber-rich, low-fat crackers such as rye Melba Toast, Triscuit Thin Crisps, and reduced-fat Wheat Thins; baked chips, "light" (with nondigestible fat) chips, or unflavored pretzels, mini graham crackers, Fig Newtons, 100% whole wheat crackers (Ak-Mak), seven grain crackers, 100% whole wheat matzoh.

## Condiments

When choosing condiments, flavor is paramount. Make sure you're aware of both calories and fat when selecting them. You'll want to barter depending on your personal choices and on how important the "true food" flavor is to you—from jams to salad dressings. A bit of sugar or fat can be a flavor plus in your product of choice, but it depends on how much you use and how often. Think low-sugar jelly versus regular jam, or reduced-fat mayonnaise versus fat-free. The choice is up to you.

### Condiments Checklist

Mustard (all varieties—check calories for certain honey mustards), ketchup, salsa, dill pickles, reduced-fat or fat-free mayonnaise, reduced-fat or fat-free Miracle Whip, low-sodium soy sauce, sriracha sauce, hot sauce, reduced-fat or fat-free salad dressing, salad dressing sprays, barbecue sauce, vegetable sprays (like Pam), dark green olive oil (first press), balsamic vinegar, rice-wine vinegar, regular jelly and jam, low-sugar jam, sugar-free jam, spreadable fruit, peanut butter (smooth or creamy—regular, not reduced fat).

## Frozen Foods

The frozen foods aisle is a fantastic aisle to shop, since it's virtually waste free. You can store foods to cook on your own terms, without worrying about short-term spoilage. From soups to breakfast foods to pizzas, meat substitutes, and frozen ice cream treats, you'll find some great calorie bargains packed with nutrients. Beware of hidden sauces loaded with extra calories and fat. Take a look at the package contents to make sure you're buying only the product, without sauce and other high-calorie add-ons (liked breaded foods to "bake" that are still loaded with calories). Limit your purchases to calorie-controlled meals, and fruits and vegetables without added sugars or fats.

## Frozen Food Checklist

*Fruits:* cherries, strawberries, blueberries, blackberries, sliced peaches, mixed berries, cut-up mango.

*Vegetables:* all varieties, without added sauce: single-variety vegetables, mixed types, for stir fry or beef stew combinations, microwaveable in bag.

*Complete Meals:* all calorie-controlled brands, chicken, beef, fish or pasta (South Beach, Lean Cuisine, Michelina's Lean, Healthy Choice, Weight Watchers), Lean Pockets, Kashi or Amy's organic meals (400 calories or less).

*Meat Substitutes/Vegetarian:* Boca Burgers (all varieties), Boca Chili, Boca Chicken Patties, Morningstar Farms soy crumbles, veggie burgers (all varieties).

*Soups:* Tabatchnik kosher soups.

*Pizza:* California Pizza Kitchen thin-crust pizza (serves three) or single-serve, Kashi Mediterranean pizza, South Beach Pizza (all varieties), Lean Pockets Pizza, Lean Cuisine French Bread Pizza.

*Breakfast Foods:* Kashi GoLean waffles, Eggo or Special K waffles, Van's waffles, VitaMuffins, VitaTops, Amy's Breakfast Burritos, calorie-controlled breakfast meals (all varieties).

*Frozen Ice Cream Treats:* Weight Watchers single-serve treats (all varieties); Skinny Cow single-serve treats; sugar-free Popsicles, single-stick Creamsicles and Popsicles (sugar-free or regular); frozen fruit bars (100% fruit); double-churned, low-fat, low-sugar ice cream (all brands); low-fat or nonfat frozen yogurt.

## Candy

The candy aisle? Am I kidding, you might ask? By now, I hope you've adopted the Real You eater's mantra that there are no bad foods, just bad portions! Make a stop in this aisle if you're looking for an occasional treat. It's not a must-do, but here are a few things you might like to have on hand.

**Candy Checklist**

Sugarless gum (all varieties), sugar-free mints and candies, Tic Tacs, Dum Dum lollipops, Tootsie Pops, single-wrapped Life Savers, single-wrapped Twizzlers licorice, 100-calorie-pack milk or dark chocolate (all varieties), Lindt dark chocolate 2 by 2 inch squares, Dove dark or milk chocolate pieces, Hershey's kisses (all varieties), mini-packs of Hot Tamales, 60-calorie Hershey's Special Dark chocolate sticks.

# 8

# Power Tools
## Weight-Loss Medications and Surgery

**If obesity really is** viewed as a chronic illness that can be managed but not cured, then why aren't there a lot of medications to treat it? I'm asked this nearly every day. First, did you ever stop to think about why it's so hard to suppress appetite? There are very few prescription medicines available for weight loss, compared to the variety of medicines used to treat chronic illnesses ranging from depression to high blood pressure, diabetes, and high cholesterol. That's because the drive to eat (the hunger signal) is hardwired in our brains for our survival. Unlike other habits like smoking, or consuming alcohol, eating is something we have to do.

Our appetite is regulated by our brain and nervous system, which is why it's really hard to find a medicine that can reduce appetite and not affect a lot of other body systems. Plus, even when a prescription medication is available, it often works for a number of weeks or months and then stops working. Why? It's because our brain always outsmarts the medicine by rerouting signals for hunger to another path. Our body is hardwired to guarantee a hunger signal, no matter what, for survival. With this principle in mind, let's take a look at some medicines that might be power tools for you. Whether it's used as a jump-start or to help sustain long-term weight loss and maintenance, a prescription medication might find its way into your toolbox.

First, there is much confusion about what's available and what really counts as a weight-loss medicine. To me, when looking at all the products out there, the lines are really blurred as to what is both safe and effective—and backed up by hard science. This really matters! Medication must always be combined with an overall long-term lifestyle plan. Avoid those tempting Internet purchases promising quick weight loss with prescription medicines, no doctor visit needed.

Evaluating medication as one of the possible power tools in your BEAM Box is not an easy task. While lifestyle is *always* the foundation of the weight-loss toolbox, it's not always enough for some people. For some of you, medication *can* help support a committed lifestyle effort, as the next step in the weight-loss treatment continuum. But what does that mean? How to choose? Does any of them work? What about over-the-counter products? I'd like to sort out all the hype and provide the help you need in deciding whether this tool belongs in your BEAM Box.

We often lump all of the pills, capsules, and other kinds of supplements into the general grouping of weight-loss medications, but there are four distinct categories—with very different safety and efficacy profiles:

> Prescription medications (FDA-approved for weight loss)
> Off-label prescription medications (FDA-approved, but not for weight loss)
> Over-the-counter medications (FDA-approved for weight loss)
> Over-the-counter dietary supplements (unregulated)

## Prescription Medications

Prescription medications are drugs that have been approved by the Food and Drug Administration (FDA) for use as weight-loss agents. They are subject to continued regulation by the FDA and are available only by prescription. They are thoroughly tested in animals and people, for both purity and safety (you won't get sick) and for efficacy (they work, but not for everyone). The FDA receives abundant evidence from the drug manufacturer and uses panels of experts to advise whether the medication meets the overall criteria of a "risk and benefit" ratio. For FDA-approved medications, the advantages must significantly outweigh any side effects of treatment. For hunger and fullness regulation, it is difficult to meet these criteria. That drive to eat is hardwired in the brain, to make sure we survive.

For weight-loss drug approval, the FDA requires an average of 5 percent weight loss, for the whole U.S. population. In other words, controlled scientific studies must document that *on average*, people lost 5 percent of their starting weight as a result of using the medication. So among the subjects of the study, some lost much more than 5 percent of their starting weight and others lost much less. For someone weighing 160 pounds, a 5 percent weight loss means a loss of at least 8 pounds. While that doesn't sound like much, it is the FDA's benchmark for an effective compound. There are also certain predictors of response that you need to discuss with your doctor to figure out if you might be a good candidate. More on that later. The main options for prescription weight-loss medication are:

**Appetite suppressants**

> *Short-term use:* phentermine (Adipex), up to twelve weeks; diethylpropion (Tenuate), up to four weeks
>
> *Long-term use:* sibutramine (Meridia), up to two years

**Fat blockers**

> *Long-term use:* orlistat (Xenical), up to two years

## Who Are They For?

You might consider prescription medications when lifestyle alone is stalled or you feel that you cannot sustain the effort level. They might even be a tool when you've lost weight and need some help in keeping it off. Begin with a discussion with your own doctor, not Dr. Google. You *can* buy medications online with a virtual prescription, but you put your health at risk. What you don't know about these medications can damage your health. All appetite-curbing medications that act on the brain, for short- or long-term use, can have negative side effects. These range from increased blood pressure and rapid heartbeat to insomnia and dry mouth.

Some medications are meant for short-term use—up to twelve weeks at a time. The long-term medications are indicated for up to two years of continuous use. While some doctors are comfortable using prescription weight-loss medications, others are not. If your doctor does not have a lot of experience with these kinds of medications, you may be referred to a physician weight-loss specialty practice or a medical center program for pharmacological treatment.

Even the FDA-approved medications don't work for everyone. Remember, only an average of 5 percent weight loss must be documented for the FDA to approve a medication. Most studies show that about one out of four people really feel it makes a lasting impact over the long term. If you want to think about adding prescription medications, your attitude going into this process must be cautiously optimistic. You should not be disappointed, or feel you did something wrong, or are a failure, if you don't get the desired result. What's most important is that medication can be worth a try *if* you have the right combination of lifestyle tools to support its use. Always keep in mind that medication can contribute to, but not *replace*, your lifestyle effort.

Unfortunately, most of these medications are not covered by insurance, so they are an out-of-pocket expense. While some can be quite pricey, if they're a workable tool to support your healthy lifestyle, they can be well worth the cost. At the very least, it's worth a chat with your doctor if you feel this might be a help.

## Appetite Suppressants

### Medicines for Short-Term Use (Up to Twelve Weeks)

There are only two prescription medications available for short-term appetite control. Both have been around for many years and are classified as "releasers," related to their chemical structure (amphetamine-like activity) and their action on the brain. The more popular of the two, phentermine, is approved for use by the FDA for up to twelve weeks. Why not longer? Good question. It's a medicine that many people like when they start it, as an answer to their dreams—"I'm not hungry"— but that only lasts for a few weeks. The effect wears off as the brain adapts to the drug, and finds other ways around the "eat less" signal, to survive. It's a strong medicine; it acts to change the *amount* of the signal one brain cell passes to another, to reduce appetite. It has a real sledgehammer effect. Phentermine is a "releaser" of more norepinephrine (a neurotransmitter) in the brain, where the greater the signal, the greater the appetite suppression. It's also a stimulant, and it provides a temporary burst of increased energy. As you might imagine, with that strong a signal, *other* brain activities are being affected as well—those that monitor blood pressure and heart rate. For many people, blood pressure and heart rate increase, and sleep patterns are interrupted.

All medications have a risk-versus-benefit profile, meaning you need to take the good with the bad regarding side effects. For some patients, with careful medical monitoring by an experienced bariatric physician, phentermine can be a short-term tool to jump-start a weight-loss plan and, in some cases, help sustain it periodically.

Another short-term appetite suppressant is diethylpropion, more commonly known by its brand name, Tenuate. Diethylpropion is another very potent drug acting on the brain; its use is limited to four weeks of continuous use. What happens after that? The medicine stops working. See what I mean? When one brain chemistry pathway blocks appetite, another pathway pops up to ensure we keep eating for survival.

Many doctors do not prescribe phentermine or diethylpropion, and with good reason. A patient must be committed to a long-term lifestyle plan and return to the doctor for regular medical monitoring. These are powerful medications, with major effects on other parts of the nervous system. If you're interested, talk to your doctor about these options, and you'll likely be referred to a bariatrician, a physician with a lot of experience with this type of medication, either in private practice or as part of a medical center program.

## Medicines for Long-Term Use (Up to Two Years)

Sibutramine (Meridia) is the only medication that has been demonstrated to moderate hunger and fullness signals in the brain that is also approved for long-term use. A complaint I often hear is that compared to the short-term drugs described above, Meridia just doesn't work very well. It often doesn't, and here's why. While the short-term drugs shout out their appetite-suppression signals, sibutramine gives a soft whisper. In contrast to phentermine or diethylpropion, Meridia does *not* release more brain neurotransmitters when a stimulation occurs. Meridia does *not* change the amount of signal that brain cells squirt out. So, while this medication does not change the amount of the chemical signal released when nerve cells communicate, it allows the normal amount of "juice" released from one brain cell to the other to stay around a bit longer and extend its effect on the surrounding brain cells. The short-term drugs release a lot more of a chemical signal very quickly. Meridia keeps the same signal your brain always has, but allows the message to stay around and act a little longer. Because of its type of action, Meridia is included in the drug class of antidepressants known as SNRIs (serotonin-norepinephrine reuptake inhibitors). Since this medication has a much smaller effect on brain chemistry, you would expect a more modest influence on hunger and fullness sensations.

With Meridia, you're still hungry for a meal but not ravenous, giving you a better sense of control before you eat. Many people tell me they are so over-hungry before a meal that they must grab something—anything—to satisfy that, and only then do they worry about making a better caloric choice. Meridia can really help if you're this type of eater. More important, Meridia has two other often reported effects: (1) it increases satiety after eating—meaning it gets you fuller, quicker, on less food; and (2) it reduces preoccupation with (constant thinking about) food.

*Melissa's Story*
## I Can't Seem to Get Full

At thirty-two, Melissa estimated she'd spent about half of her life concerned with her weight. Since she'd started college, her weight had been creeping up slowly and consistently. She agreed that the college party life contributed 25 pounds in four years, and that was her new normal after graduation. Now, a decade later, with a relatively sedentary lifestyle as a computer programmer, Melissa found herself another 20 pounds heavier, despite a commitment to healthier eating. The weight just "snuck up on me," she said. On a five-foot-three-inch frame, those 45 pounds put her at a BMI of 33. Yet, while she did not have a medical illness, she was shocked to find that she fell into the medically obese category and was slightly panicked about what to do.

Her first step was to build a BEAM Box with the right combination of eating, activity, and behavioral tools. Melissa's goal was to get in touch with her inability to stay on track, which had resulted in persistent weight creep. After staying with her plan for eight weeks, Melissa did lose 8 pounds, but felt she was already struggling. She was honest in her assessment that her effort level was maxed out, and she needed another tool to help. In addition, as Melissa tracked her hunger fullness ratings over the past two months, she felt that it was becoming increasingly difficult to both sense her Level 2 of fullness (contentment without being stuffed—see the Fernstrom Fundamentals in chapter 3) and not eat through that signal.

Melissa met the medical criteria for a trial of Meridia, and her primary care doctor agreed to a one-month test period, with a blood pressure check at the end of two weeks. Melissa tolerated the daily Meridia capsule (10 mg) very well. She had minimal side effects—her blood pressure was unchanged, and she reported only a bit of a dry mouth, which she resolved by drinking more water. After about three days on the medicine, Melissa noticed that she felt more content with less food. She was able to stop, and end a meal leaving food on her plate. "This felt like a very natural thing to me," she added, and actually wondered if the medication was working, since she didn't feel "revved up." Melissa felt that her hunger and fullness thermostat had been slightly readjusted, allowing her to eat about 500 fewer calories a day with moderate, but not heroic, effort. Melissa's rate of weight loss went from a pound a week to 2 pounds a week during her first month on Meridia—she lost 8 additional pounds in one month while taking Meridia. In addition, Melissa had the relief of not having food "constantly on my mind," and was able to commit to a thirty-five-minute brisk walk daily. Melissa remained on Meridia for another six months and lost an additional 30 pounds, for a total of 46 pounds.

Meridia continues to be a useful tool for Melissa for weight maintenance. Now on Meridia for one year, she has maintained her 45-pound
weight loss. Since her response to Meridia has been a big help, and far
beyond the average, she will remain on the drug for another year, to support her weight stability. Melissa is confident that when she goes off the
Meridia (at the end of two years), she will have mastered and ingrained
the lifestyle skills to help her compensate for her biological vulnerability.
With her doctor's support, she understands that she may need to return
to this power tool on an intermittent basis to help support her lifestyle
effort in the future.

## Fat Blockers

Some people don't struggle with hunger and fullness management, yet
they find it hard to limit fat intake. Or they might not be medical candidates for a drug that acts on the brain, because the side effects are a
health risk (that's why you *must* see your own doctor before considering *any* weight loss medication). Here's where a prescription fat blocker
comes in. What does it block, exactly, you might ask? Fat that you eat?
Yes. Fat already in your body? No!

Orlistat (Xenical) is what's called a "pancreatic lipase inhibitor."
A simple way to think of this medicine is that it blocks the breakdown
and absorption of about a third of the fat you eat at each meal (you take
this three times a day, before each meal). It *only* blocks fat absorption,
and if you eat extra protein or carbohydrate calories, that's not affected.
Because it blocks fat calories, the recommendation is to keep your fat
intake at each meal at 30 percent of calories or below (that's 100 calories,
or about 10 grams of fat for a 300-calorie meal), to avoid too much fat
being eliminated at one time.

A major complaint with Xenical is that the side effects are "gross."
Now, the side effects that people complain about are diarrhea, bloating, and gas. To set the record straight, they are not side effects but
what the drug actually does. If you are experiencing these symptoms,
that means the drug is working and you've eaten too much fat at one

meal. Managing these effects is part of the learning curve of using Xenical (or its FDA-approved sister compound, Alli, described below. Alli is a lower dose of this medication, available over the counter without a prescription). Here are a few questions to help you identify if Xenical is worth a try for you:

Do you struggle with controlling your fat intake?

Do you have a hard time identifying hidden fats in food?

Do you do a lot of restaurant eating?

Do you need "negative reinforcement" (a negative action) of a medicine to actually feel it working?

If you've answered yes to two or more questions, than you might give it a try. Start with a visit to your primary care doctor, or consider the over-the-counter version, Alli (see "Over-the-Counter Products" on page 177).

## How to Talk to Your Doctor about Prescription Medication

Don't be afraid to open a discussion with your doctor about weight-loss medications. Your primary care doctor is always the best place to start. If your own doctor is not comfortable with prescribing without a structured lifestyle plan in place, you can at least get a referral to a medical-center-based comprehensive program, or a board-certified bariatrician (weight-loss physician), or a similar medically supervised plan that supports the toolbox approach.

Have a list of questions prepared, and think about how a particular kind of medication might work for you. There are medical guidelines for prescription drugs, starting with body mass index, your height-to-weight ratio that reflects health risk. (BMI is described in appendix A, and you can check out the chart there.)

There are two ways to meet the first medical criteria: (1) you have a BMI of 30 or higher; or (2) you have a BMI of 27 or higher, with a significant medical illness, such as diabetes, high blood pressure, or elevated cholesterol. If you qualify, then it's an individual decision between you and your doctor which medication to try.

You'll also want to make sure your doctor discusses the pros and cons of *your specific health* profile. You might be a candidate for one medicine but not another. It's hard to know for sure the predictors of medication response, as all the published studies show a huge amount of variation—from no loss to dozens of pounds.

## Be Aware of Medications That Can Cause Weight Gain

Even if you're not a candidate for weight-loss medication, you'll want to review with your doctor your present medication profile, to determine if you're taking any medication that could be packing on some pounds as a side effect of its primary use. While the mechanism of action is not well understood for all these drugs, they act to either increase hunger, reduce metabolic rate, or some combination of the two. Either way, the result is an excess of calories, stored as extra pounds. Here's a list of the categories you want to review with your doctor, to see if a substitution might be appropriate.

### Mental Health Treatment

Tricyclic antidepressants (Elavil, Tofranil, Pamelor, Remeron)
SSRI antidepressants (Paxil, Zoloft, Luvox)
Antipsychotics (Haldol, Clorazil, Zyprexa, Risperdol)
Anticonvulsants (Depakote, Tegretol, Neurontin)

### Diabetes Treatment

Sulfonylureas (Glucotrol, Glynase)
Thiazolidenediones (Actos, Avandia)
Insulin (Humulog)

### Inflammation Treatment

Corticosteroids (Cortisone)

### Blood Pressure Treatment

Beta-blockers (Tenormin, Inderal, Toprol)

Note: If you've been taking a medication for longer than six months without a change in weight, and you start to notice weight gain *after* that, it's unlikely that the medication is the cause. Weight gain as a side effect is usually noticed during the early weeks of starting a new medication. Either way, talk to your doctor if you suspect that your medication might be making your lifestyle effort more difficult. The good news is that weight gained as a side effect of medication is no more difficult to lose than any other kind of weight.

## Realistic Expectations

I'm often asked about what to expect with weight-loss medications. My answer is always the same. If you identify your eating barriers, and one of these medications seems like it might help support the lifestyle effort, it's worth a try to add this power tool to your toolbox. Since response rates for *all* of these medications range from zero pounds to more than 100 pounds lost, it's impossible to predict whom it will help. Cautious optimism is in order, and if you don't try, you don't know. If these don't work for you, *it's not your fault.* You wouldn't blame yourself if a blood pressure medicine didn't work for you, you'd just switch to a different medicine. Not so easy with weight-loss drugs, when there are so few options. Pharmacologic treatment of obesity is still in its infancy, and while there are limited medication options right now, a number of possible future drugs are under study (see "The Future of Prescription Weight-Loss Drugs" on page 176).

# "Off-Label" Prescription Medications

Here's a category of weight-loss medications that causes real confusion. It's a prescription medicine, so that's all good, right? What does "off-label" mean? The term refers to medications that are approved for use by the FDA for another treatment—not weight loss. Just as some medications promote weight gain as a side effect, such as those described above, other medications have the opposite effect. There are several medications with the side effects of appetite suppression, weight loss, or both. Most of the evidence suggesting these drugs work for weight loss comes from observing patients taking the medication for the approved use. For example, the antiseizure medication Topamax is often associated with unintended weight loss in patients being treated for epilepsy. In this case, the side effect is severe appetite suppression.

### Some Off-Label Drugs Used for Weight Loss

Topamax (approved to treat seizures and migraine headaches)
Glucophage and Byetta (approved for treatment of diabetes)
Wellbutrin (approved for treatment of depression)
Adderall and Ritalin (approved for attention deficit hyperactivity disorder)
Provigil (approved for chronic fatigue and sleep disorders)

Those people being treated for disease have reported a variety of effects from this drug group, ranging from a reduction in appetite and fewer food cravings to great energy and less focus on food. There are no scientific studies showing these drugs are effective for weight loss, and you can put yourself at risk for damaging side effects for such an off-label use. The negative side effects are not worth the risk.

Right now, most physicians will not prescribe these drugs for weight loss, but a small group of physicians actually support and encourage this use. While the pharmaceutical companies producing these medications do *not* support the off-label use, some are working to modify the original formula to develop a weight-loss drug for the future. Still, this does not stop many people from looking for these alternatives. Whether used alone or in weight-loss cocktails, these can be medically quite risky. Talk with your own doctor or contact a weight-loss specialist for a more in-depth discussion.

## The Future of Prescription Weight-Loss Drugs: What's on the Horizon?

You've gotten the message by now that it's really hard to develop medications that affect hunger and fullness without causing a lot of negative side effects. The good news is that some pharmaceutical companies are working toward developing new drugs with few side effects, as well as forms of off-label medications that might be safe and effective specifically for weight loss. The bottom line is that appetite-suppressing medications, even the newer ones under study, seem to work well for some people, but only for about six to nine months, and then they help support weight maintenance, with no further weight-loss effect.

Even after years of study, the approval process can be daunting. Over the past few years, there seemed to be great initial promise for a medication called rimonabant (Zimulti in Canada). This medicine acts on the brain to block hunger signals produced by brain chemicals that are found in a brain pathway called the "endocannabinoid" system. Does this word kind of sound familiar? Yes, it's related to the same group of brain cells that marijuana (cannabis) acts on. There's been a lot of interest in this medicine, since many people understand the mechanism of action. Marijuana enhances the action of this group of brain cells and provides an increased sense of well-being and mood improvement, as well as appetite stimulation. In contrast, rimonabant *blocks* this action and suppresses appetite. It also, as a side effect on mood, can cause the opposite effect of marijuana: it can produce depressive symptoms in some people. This remains a controversial medication. Never approved for use in the United States, the drug was recently removed from the European market, and its risk/benefit profile continues to be debated.

While there are other experimental drugs in the development pipeline, including the use of low-dose drug combinations of "off label" weight-loss drugs, the approval process for both safety and efficacy in the United States is long. For now, the field of prescription weight loss drugs is still in its infancy.

## Over-the-Counter Products

To use or not to use—that is the question. Over-the-counter products have great appeal, because they help you keep a certain distance from your health-care provider. That can be both good and bad for your general health and well-being. For many people, being able to purchase the promise of a product without permission, prescription, or judgment provides a sense of control and empowerment. It can also introduce some health risk. A note of caution before you enter this uncharted territory. Check with your primary care doctor, or local pharmacist, before trying an unregulated product, particularly if the product is described as an "appetite suppressant" or a "fat burner."

It's appealing to be able to obtain a product with no medical supervision involved. It seems to provide us with more choice, but this is simply an illusion. There is currently no over-the-counter medication with FDA approval to support the claims of either suppressing appetite or burning more fat.

## FDA-Approved Dietary Supplements

There is one product that has FDA approval for over-the-counter use. Marketed under the brand name Alli, it acts as a partial fat blocker, and is the over-the-counter version of the prescription drug Xenical. Similar to other available over-the-counter versions of prescription medications, Alli is half the dose of the prescription-strength drug. You can purchase Alli without consulting a health professional, but it's always a good idea to discuss adding any new weight-loss tools with your doctor.

Like Xenical, Alli blocks the absorption of some of the fat that is ingested at meals. It has no action on the brain to moderate hunger and fullness, but it can help to save calories by blocking one-fourth of the fat eaten in each meal (the prescription version, Xenical, blocks one-third of the fat at each meal). Translated into calories, this might help you lose up to 50 percent *more* weight than you would expect with lifestyle changes alone. Alli only acts on fat calories consumed and has no effect on the absorption of protein or carbohydrates, so if you consume more of these, Alli will not make a difference.

With any fat blocker, it's important to monitor fat intake closely. Remember, Alli will block about one-fourth of the fat eaten at each meal. So if you eat 20 grams of fat, it will block 5 grams (45 calories); if you eat 60 grams at a meal, it will block 15 grams (135 calories). It's recommended that you consume no more than 30 percent of daily calories from fat at each meal in order to avoid *too* much fat blockage, resulting in unpleasant digestive effects like gas, bloating, and diarrhea. When I hear complaints about these bad side effects of Alli, I tell my patients that this is actually the *main* effect, it's just that they are consuming too much fat. If you're experiencing these side effects, revisit your food intake and eliminate some sources of hidden fat.

## *Gloria's Story*
## I Need Immediate Reinforcement

Gloria, a forty-five-year-old administrator, had always struggled with an extra 40 pounds, and knew her problem. "I love rich foods," she said. Having grown up in South Carolina and relocated to Pennsylvania, she yearned for the wonderful comfort foods of home. Whether cooking at home for friends or eating in restaurants, Gloria told me, her "fat tooth" was always around to sabotage her efforts. While in the past she had tried for years to cut down her fat, there was never any consequence to her actions, she said. "I need something to keep me honest," she added.

Gloria was looking for a power tool to help her better manage her high fat consumption. Gloria's BEAM Box was in great shape, with tools for how to eat, move, and manage stress; but lack of consistency was the problem. She was managing well with her plan most days, but felt she could make much better choices with her frequent restaurant meals and on special occasions, which seemed to be at least once a week. Her present plan allowed her to stay even and not gain—still a plus. That was not satisfactory for her, as she had recently been diagnosed with high cholesterol, and her doctor told her if she could not change her dietary habits and lose some weight in the next six months, he would recommend that she take a cholesterol-lowering medication.

Gloria did not want to pursue the medication route as a next step, and so used a combination of lifestyle and Alli to keep her on a daily track of a low-fat intake. She took Alli three times daily before meals to make sure she kept her fat intake at 30 percent of calories or below. Gloria didn't fool herself by reserving Alli for when she felt confident in her food choice. She took Alli before every meal to ensure she would stay on track and eat a low-fat meal or else suffer the consequences of intestinal disturbances. In fact, this is what Gloria liked about taking Alli. "It does keep me honest." Her restaurant eating improved, and she always ordered a main dish salad, or plain grilled fish or chicken with dressing on the side. Even in a fast-food restaurant where she went with her nephews once a week, she ordered a main dish salad without dressing (she used fresh lemon), and a small bowl of chili (skipping the cheese and sour cream).

For Gloria, Alli was an important tool. With her effort now more consistent, she went from being weight stable with moderate effort to losing 5 to 6 pounds each month, consistently, for the next six months, for a total of 37 pounds. Now weight stable, Gloria still takes Alli every day to remain on track. As she told me, she'll know when the time may be right to discontinue it; but for now, she's including it as a permanent tool to help support her lifestyle for long-term weight stability.

---

As with prescription-strength Xenical, it's pretty easy to figure out if Alli might be a useful power tool for you. The same four basic questions apply:

Do you struggle with controlling your fat intake?

Do you have a hard time identifying hidden fats in food?

Do you do a lot of restaurant eating?

Do you need "negative reinforcement" (a negative action) of a medicine to actually feel it working?

If you answered yes to two or more of these questions, Alli might be the boost you need. And, even though you can get it over the counter, it's always a good idea to check with your doctor before starting.

## Unregulated Dietary Supplements

Many millions of dollars are spent each year on weight-loss supplements. The promise of effortless and quick weight loss is too hard to pass up. There's a lot of confusion here, and with good reason. Many of these products do contain active ingredients found in nature. But natural doesn't always mean safe. Arsenic, a potent poison, is also natural! It's really not surprising in nature to find compounds that arouse, sedate, and suppress appetite as part of the rhythm of life. The problem is, none of these products is regulated at all by the FDA or any governmental agency, even though many are packaged to look like medications.

Whether a product is termed a "fat burner" or an "appetite suppressant," be wary of these claims. Because there is no regulation of dietary supplements by any official government agency, there is an abundance of products on the market with no documented evidence of efficacy, safety, or purity. This lack of regulation comes from the Dietary Supplements Health and Education Act (DSHEA), which was passed by Congress in 1994. The act allowed any product originating from a plant source to be sold to the consumer without any oversight by the FDA or other national regulatory agencies. So documentation of efficacy, safety, and purity remained in the hands of individual companies.

Only if a compound can be shown to be harmful, as was the case with the widely used plant compound ephedra (ma-huang), is the FDA authorized to remove it from the marketplace. While the biological efficacy of ephedra was never in question, the variability in purity and dosage posed a continuing health risk, documented by significant illness and death. The FDA removed ephedra from the market as a weight-loss supplement in 2006. Many currently popular supplements contain stimulants, such as caffeine and guarana (a plant product similar to caffeine), or other less well-known compounds, such as bitter orange.

At the very least, these products are a waste of money (they can be quite expensive); at the worst, they can have contaminants or cause side effects such as stimulant effects on your cardiovascular system, which can result in serious health damage or even death. Because of the variability in purity and dosage, always let your doctor know what you're taking, particularly if you take other prescription medications. Beware of sensational claims. When it comes to weight-loss supplements, if it sounds too good to be true, it probably is.

**Weight-Loss Supplement Red Flags**

- Money-back guarantee
- Guaranteed quick weight loss without effort
- Claims of "similar results to a prescription medication"
- Claims of "natural" weight-loss compounds
- Claims based on a single scientific study
- Personal testimonials of "success"
- Limited (or no) expectation of lifestyle change

# Weight-Loss Surgery

Weight-loss (bariatric) surgery can be a positive, life-altering power tool for the right person. The hardest part is determining if it's the right tool for you. Lifestyle is always the foundation of weight loss, and surgery might be a tool to support the lifestyle effort (and make it easier) but not to replace it. There are many pros and cons to weight-loss surgery, but inaccurate personal opinions often muddy the weight-loss surgery waters. You may already know people who swear that surgery was the best thing they ever did, as well as others who curse the day they even considered it.

The benefits can be life-changing because it's not just the large amount of weight that can be lost (about 70 percent of the extra—or 70 pounds for someone needing to lose 100 pounds); it's the mental boost of knowing that this weight loss can finally be sustained with reasonable lifestyle effort. No more yo-yo syndrome or major weight excursions. While this sounds like the perfect plan if you've got 100 pounds or more to lose, it's important to emphasize that this is major surgery (including general anesthesia), and major surgery always comes with a risk. It's figuring out if the risk/benefit ratio is one that works for you that's important.

With any surgery, there is always a small risk of death, and with obesity surgery it's around one in a hundred people (or even less)—no different from other major surgery that requires general anesthesia. There can be medical complications from the procedure, as well as postoperative medical and lifestyle concerns that need to be evaluated. So, while the benefits can be tremendously health promoting, it's important to make this decision in a methodical way and compile a list of both the pros and cons for your own health history.

Weight-loss surgery has been well documented to help people both lose weight and keep it off for the long term. In our country, we're really good at taking weight off but not very good at keeping it off—and that's where surgery *might* be in the cards for you. Obesity surgery is not a quick fix for anyone, yet it can make the lifestyle effort less of a struggle, with a bigger weight loss "payoff" for consistent effort. That is a huge mental boost. But don't be fooled—the lifestyle effort *after* weight loss surgery is more challenging than *any* nonsurgical lifestyle plan can ever be. Why? Because you can't decide you'd like to go off the plan and coast for a while. Once you make the commitment to obesity surgery, it's a commitment for life.

Whether surgery might be a good tool for you is a loaded question, with multiple answers. While obesity surgery can be a missing tool for thousands of people every year, it's a decision that takes a lot of information gathering and a lot of soul searching. The benefits are significant for the right person: (1) long-term weight loss and maintenance; (2) improvement or cure of existing medical conditions; (3) reduction or elimination of prescription medications. Read on to see if surgery is right for you.

## When to Consider Obesity Surgery

Before considering weight-loss surgery, you must be absolutely sure you are doing it for the right reasons. You *cannot* view it as a "last ditch" effort to lose weight, or do it because "nothing works and I need something." If you have that mind-set, I can assure you, you're setting yourself up for disappointment. You need to go into this process understanding that surgery will support, but not replace, your lifestyle effort. Translated into daily living, this tool allows you to eat around 1,200 to 1,500 calories a day (in the long run), without feeling like you're starving to death.

Obesity surgery can be a good choice if you feel your hunger and fullness thermostat is set too high. This is biology, not behavior. The most frequent comments I hear from surgical candidates are that "I never feel full," or "I can't remember a time that I didn't need much more food than anyone around me to fill me up." For the right person, the control over food that was so elusive in the past becomes more manageable. You will still need to make a daily effort to maintain a healthy lifestyle, but the effort will produce a great payoff in both short- and long-term weight loss.

Weight-loss surgery will definitely help you consume fewer calories (your anatomy is changed), but your reasons for eating do not change. Here's where behavioral tools are key. If you're considering surgery, you will discover ways to manage stress that do not involve food, and learn to live in a world where food is everywhere and available twenty-four hours a day. If this sounds like you, read on.

To help you get started, take Fernstrom's Surgical Readiness Quiz. If you can answer yes to all the questions, you're off to a good start. These are the ten key points to understand when you take the surgical path.

### Fernstrom's Surgical Readiness Quiz

- Do you accept partial responsibility for your weight gain?
- Are you willing to work on regaining control of your food intake?
- Are you willing to confront your eating sabotages?
- Are you comfortable with managing the stress of long-term food restriction?
- Do you have realistic expectations of weight-loss surgery?
- Are you prepared for the regimentation of the postsurgical lifestyle?
- Are you willing to become more physically active every day?
- Are you willing to meet with someone (or a group) for ongoing support?
- Are you willing to be in a follow-up program for life?
- Are you willing to seek additional help when needed?

## *Jennifer's Story*
# I Want to Have a Baby

At twenty-seven years old, Jennifer couldn't remember a time when she wasn't heavy. "I was always the biggest girl in the class," she candidly told me. While she recalled some painful teasing, starting in elementary school, Jennifer had had a lot of friends and was a happy teenager. "My friends didn't care that I'm fat," she said. She came from a large, close-knit family that celebrated all occasions large and small with an abundance of food. "Food is love in my family," she said. In her teens, Jennifer didn't have any health problems related to her weight, but she recalled that her periods were irregular, and she often missed several months at a time. She felt it would probably straighten out over time.

Jennifer couldn't remember a time when she wasn't on a diet, and on some diets she would lose as much as 50 pounds before gaining it all back after she "stopped trying." This pattern went on for several years. Jennifer met Ted in college, and they were married three years after graduating from college. At that time, Jennifer's weight was 240 pounds. On her five-foot-two-inch frame, that gave her a BMI of 44. Jennifer and Ted wanted to start a family. After a year of trying without becoming pregnant, even knowing that her menstrual cycle was not always regular, Jennifer talked with her gynecologist about what could be wrong. Her doctor explained that obesity is a major factor relating to infertility. With a lifelong history of obesity, and many failed attempts with lifestyle alone for weight control, Jennifer felt a surgical option would help her get the weight off faster, in a safe manner, and would help her maintain lifelong control. She was through with crash diets. Her plan was straightforward. She had multiple tools for eating and activity already in her BEAM Box, and had discussed a surgical option with her primary care doctor. She was evaluated for gastric banding, and met all the criteria. After a six-month lifestyle monitoring period (required by her insurance company; she had optimized her lifestyle plan by month five), Jennifer went for her banding surgery. Her goal of weighing 160 pounds (an 80-pound loss) was reached after eighteen months. Her BEAM Box and yearly follow-up with her surgeon and primary care doctor remain firmly in place. Jennifer resumed monthly periods and happily became pregnant two years after her banding surgery. She and Ted are now the proud parents of a baby daughter, and Jennifer is confident that she can maintain her healthy lifestyle and weight with the help of a band. She is committed to healthy eating and activity for her whole family. "I know my daughter won't struggle the way I did," she added.

---

## Are You a Surgical Candidate?

Obesity surgery is considered elective surgery, meaning that it's your choice to consider but it may not always be medically recommended. While a lot of accurate information is available online, none of it is specific to you. You'll want to discuss this option with your primary care doctor, who needs to be supportive of your effort and willing to discuss the pros and cons relating to your personal health. A discussion of whether you meet the criteria for surgery is the first step. National guidelines are already in place.

First, determine your BMI (see appendix A). If your number is 40 or higher, you meet the excess pounds criterion for surgery, even if you have no medical illnesses relating to your weight. Many programs also have age limitations, though, so if you're under eighteen, or over sixty-five, a BMI of 40 or higher does not automatically make you a candidate. If your BMI is higher than 60, or you have significant medical problems (such as uncontrolled blood pressure or diabetes), you may need further medical evaluation and care before you can follow the surgical path.

### Medical Criteria for Weight-Loss Surgery

- BMI of 40 or higher (no documented medical illness)
- BMI of 35 to 39.9 (documented significant medical illness)
- Ability to tolerate general anesthesia
- Weight roughly 80 to 100 pounds over predicted healthy weight
- Documented history of failed lifestyle weight loss
- Recent (six-month) documentation of medically supervised lifestyle
- Commitment to healthy eating and regular physical activity

The decision to consider obesity surgery is a complex one, loaded with many factors. People often misinterpret the decision to pursue surgery as the biggest challenge. In fact, it's the first of many steps. The best attitude with which to begin the obesity surgery path is *patience*. The time that passes after you first decide that surgery might be a good tool for you until you're finally in the operating room can vary by many months. For some, it can be as short as several months, while for others, it can be a year or more.

**First Three Steps toward Obesity Surgery**

1. See if you meet the medical/surgical criteria (see above).
2. Check with your insurance company for specific operations and services that are covered, and for required out-of-pocket expenses and copayments (or consider a self-pay option).
3. Find a surgeon. (See "Finding a Surgeon" on page 189.)

*Sheila's Success Story*
## Too Late for Me?

When she first came to see me, Sheila thought it was too late for her to get control of her weight. To structure her program and build her BEAM Box, we went way back in time for some insights. At fifty-eight, Sheila could not recall a time that she had ever been totally happy with her weight, but acknowledged that until she had children, she had managed to stay in a size 10. When her clothes began to feel tight, she resisted the urge to get a few outfits to tide her over until she was back to her old size. That was more than twenty years earlier. With her first pregnancy, Sheila gained 70 pounds, and even after trying to get back to her prepregnancy weight, she was stalled with an extra 45 pounds. Two more pregnancies followed, and while Sheila paid more attention to her lifestyle, and gained about 50 pounds with each pregnancy, she wound up with another 40 pounds after those two pregnancies. By the end of her childbearing years, Sheila was 85 pounds heavier than her size 10. "My husband always told me he loved me no matter what size package I was in," she added.

One year later, Sheila's weight was still creeping up slowly, and she found herself 10 pounds heavier than she had been the year before. Now she was 95 pounds heavier than in her size 10 days. She was frightened by a recent visit to her doctor, where she was diagnosed with high blood pressure and type 2 diabetes. "Your weight has finally caught up to your health," her doctor told her. "I can't believe this happened," she said. "And to think that I was complaining when I was a size 10!"

Sheila had a cousin who had undergone gastric banding about two years earlier, and was doing well. "Would surgery be an option?" she first asked. Sheila did meet the surgical criteria, but agreed she was not ready to take that step until she could demonstrate to herself that she had the long-term commitment to a challenging lifestyle. She felt defeated and was unsure how to begin. The first goal with her plan was to stop the weight creep, with her goal being to just not gain. That took the pressure off her "performance." For six months, we built a BEAM Box that provided structured meals, riding on a recumbent bike, and working with her doctor to select medications for her blood pressure and diabetes that didn't promote weight gain or make it harder to lose weight.

At the end of six months, she was surprised to see that not only had she maintained her weight and stopped the creep, she had lost 15 pounds. At this point of reevaluation, despite a consistent and devoted lifestyle change, Sheila felt she needed to add the surgical tool to continue her weight loss. Sheila was evaluated for surgery, and she and her surgeon agreed on a stomach banding. Sheila understood that the rate of weight loss from banding was slow and steady, compared with the results from bypass, but she was close to her cousin who had done so well with the banding and had a lot of support from her. Sheila's banding went well, and she went on to lose 60 pounds in the next fifteen months. Combined with the 15 pounds she lost prior to surgery, Sheila took off a total of 75 pounds and has been able to keep them off for the past four years. Her high blood pressure and diabetes are gone, and she feels great. She is back to shopping for size 10 clothes. Sheila looks and feels great, and her husband and three sons are thrilled to see how happy and healthy she is.

## Insurance Issues

You might assume that your insurance company will cover all costs for obesity surgery. It's necessary—right? Yes and no. Since obesity surgery falls into what's considered the elective surgery category, it's often a toss-up. It's not a safe bet to assume that your insurance company will cover this service, so you've got to make that call. You need to find out which kinds of surgery are covered in your plan, and whether you're responsible for some of the associated costs, or for a specific copay for the total amount. Every plan is different, so call ahead. Most plans also require at least six months of physician-supervised lifestyle documentation, separate nutrition education, and psychological assessment as part of the preoperative workup. Your surgeon can help coordinate this process.

What if your plan does *not* cover weight-loss surgery? Many people find themselves in an unhappy position when their surgeon supports their surgical option but their insurance company does not cover it, or they are denied approval for a variety of reasons. While your surgeon can help you appeal a negative decision, you can also consider the self-pay option. Nationwide comprehensive packages are often available. The self-pay comprehensive costs of weight-loss surgery are about the same investment as buying a new car. In fact, if you look at it like a car loan, your car usually lasts less than a decade. This operation is an investment in your life that will keep giving you the gift of good health. Only you can decide the value of lifelong improved health. Low-interest financing is often available, and the surgical program you attend will have a staff member who can help you with this.

## Finding a Surgeon

You first want to make sure you see a surgeon with specific experience in bariatric surgery. It's important to select both a surgeon and a hospital that are accredited as a Center of Excellence by the American Society of Metabolic and Bariatric Surgery, the American College of Surgery, or other accreditations your insurance company will accept. Even if you have a referral from a friend or your family doctor (often a good way to locate a bariatric surgeon), ask for your surgeon's specific credentials when calling for an appointment. Studies show that the greater the experience of both the surgeon and the hospital, the better the outcome. It's the reason most insurance companies now will only pay for surgeries that are done at accredited Centers of Excellence, which go through a comprehensive certification process covering everything from lifestyle programs to anesthesia care, operating rooms and staffing, and surgical care.

Before your first visit with the surgeon, it's a good idea to give some thought to the kind of operation you think is a good match. But at your visit, be willing to hear the surgeon's point of view about your best long-term options. Two of the most frequently done operations are the lap band (stomach-size restriction only, so you eat less) and the gastric bypass (stomach-size restriction plus mild calorie malabsorption).

**Types of Weight-Loss Surgery**

1. Restriction procedures make the stomach smaller.
2. Malabsorption procedures block calories from being absorbed.
3. Combination procedures result in both a smaller stomach and fewer calories absorbed.

There are several different types of weight-loss operations to change your anatomy, so you can pick one tailored to your own needs. The surgical treatment of obesity has more than half a century of research and development. The earliest operations were much cruder and could have truly awful side effects, but the newest surgical techniques are sophisticated, much safer, and provide a superior "risk/benefit" ratio. If you choose to move ahead with this power tool, the decision to do so is ultimately your own. However, establishing the best type of surgical solution truly is a process of mutual trust between you and your bariatric surgeon.

## Restriction Procedures

### Gastric Banding

Enter the newest and most improved stomach restriction surgery. Called the "laparoscopic adjustable band," gastric banding has essentially replaced the older stomach stapling procedure. A silicone belt is surgically placed around the stomach. A long connector tube goes from the band to a port attached just under the rib cage, to allow long-term adjustments to maintain the original tightness of the band. This port is small, and it is placed under the skin, so you don't see it, but the surgeon can locate it and feel it when the band needs to be adjusted. Over a period of months, you adapt to a new sense of fullness from consuming far fewer calories than it took before to provide contentment. Your stomach is now about the size of an egg, rather than the size of a quart of milk. That makes sense when you visualize what the actual operation is designed to do.

After the surgery, both lifestyle and surgical follow-up are needed, with close monitoring of both for the first year. Weight loss is slow and steady, with about 50 to 70 percent of your extra weight gone within two years. That means if you need to lose 100 pounds, you can expect to lose about 50 to 70 pounds, with extra support from the band. The total loss varies from person to person, depending on lifestyle effort; you might lose more or less than the predicted average.

Close follow-up with the surgeon is needed, to help monitor the lifestyle effort, rate of weight loss, and sense of hunger and fullness provided by the band. The band can be tightened to cut down on food intake, if needed. The adjustment is done via the small port secured in the original surgery. A small amount of sterile saltwater is injected into the port (it doesn't hurt), which then stiffens and tightens the band slightly. During the first year, adjustments are frequent, until you reach a reasonable balance between your lifestyle effort and continued weight loss. It's important to understand that the band does not *replace* the lifestyle effort, but just helps to make it easier (see "Lifestyle Tools after Surgery" on page 195). Always review your personal risks and benefits with your surgeon and primary care doctor.

## Gastroplasty

Most people are familiar with gastroplasty, which is popularly known as "stomach stapling." This old restriction procedure is rarely performed nowadays, because newer techniques are more effective. In gastroplasty, surgical staples are used to make the stomach smaller, but the stomach is a muscle, which can stretch over time. When someone eats more food over a period of time, the stomach pouch stretches like a balloon, and can often even interrupt the staple line. So, while the short-term results of this surgery can be promising, weight regain is usually a sure thing. Since most patients regain all of their lost weight (even up to 100 pounds), this procedure is usually discouraged as an option.

## Malabsorption Procedures

### Jejuno-Ileal Bypass

There are also operations that don't alter the size of your stomach. They allow you to still eat a lot of food, but they greatly reduce the ability of calories to be absorbed into your body. No absorption of calories, no extra calories stored as fat. Sounds like a dream, right? A highly popular surgery several decades ago, the jejuno-ileal bypass, or JI bypass, kept your stomach size intact but blocked the calories from being absorbed. This is what many people incorrectly think about when first hearing about weight-loss surgery. You may have heard stories from friends or relatives, or seen them online, of people who had this operation many years ago. The problem with this procedure is that no behaviors are forced to change—you can still eat the same amount, but very little is digested, with huge metabolic consequences. Unless a major lifestyle change is implemented, protein and vitamin/mineral deficiencies often occur after this type of severe surgery, along with a lot of digestive problems, including severe diarrhea and dehydration. Nowadays this surgery, or a variation, is used only in the most severe types of obesity, and only after careful evaluation on a case-by-case basis. Because of the long-term health problems associated with this type of surgery, many insurance companies no longer cover it.

## Combination Procedures

### Roux-en-y Gastric Bypass

The surgical research community has moved ahead to develop what is often referred to as the gold standard of obesity surgery, the gastric bypass. This combines the process of creating a smaller stomach (restriction) with some bypassing of intestinal digestion of calories (mild malabsorption) — the best of both worlds of an anatomic change.

In gastric bypass surgery, a small stomach pouch is surgically created — initially the size of your pinky, which over time stretches to about the size of an egg. The stomach is physically separated, and the small pouch becomes your new stomach. I'm often asked what happens to the rest of your big stomach — is it removed? Absolutely not! You need the remaining stomach in place, to continue to produce and release digestive juices. It remains safe, and is in a sterile environment in your body, but it just doesn't fill up with food.

The small pouch gives a much earlier signal for satiety — of course, since it can't hold much food! So how is this different from the band, and a restriction operation? Here's where the mild calorie blockage comes in. In a gastric bypass, after food leaves your stomach, it is rerouted to a lower part of your intestine — literally bypassing some of the calorie absorption part of the digestive tract. You are still absorbing calories and nutrients, but further down in the digestive tract, so there is less capacity of your intestines to absorb the food (the bypassed part). The result is that fewer calories are eaten; and of those calories, fewer are absorbed. It's kind of a "one-two punch" when it comes to obesity surgery.

For the right person, this operation can have amazing results. The outcomes for those who really comply with the lifestyle plan are tremendous — about 70 to 80 percent of excess weight is lost. The loss is relatively rapid — much quicker than with restriction alone, which makes sense. It takes roughly twelve months to lose about 100 pounds, but it can be faster or slower depending on your starting weight and lifestyle effort. That means, if you needed to lose 100 pounds, you could expect to lose about 80 pounds with help from the operation. The big *if* is the lifestyle commitment.

### *Michael's (Continuing) Story*
### Adding a Power Tool

You may remember Michael (and his wife, Nikki) from chapter 6. Building his BEAM Box began with a visit to his primary care doctor. He had 150 pounds to lose, and multiple medical problems related to his weight.

His high blood pressure and elevated cholesterol were under control with medication, but at thirty-six, he did not want to be taking medication forever. With the diagnosis of sleep apnea, and nightly treatment with a C-PAP apparatus, Michael now was sleeping soundly and his fatigue was greatly reduced. He was highly motivated and energized to permanently alter his lifestyle.

Michael faced the difficult challenge of taking back control of a lifestyle that had no structure. He realized he had a long journey ahead of him with more than 100 pounds to lose. Lifestyle would always be his foundation, he knew, but he *might* need to consider a power tool, if lifestyle alone could not produce or sustain the weight loss needed for good health. He agreed to a six-month plan of lifestyle change, to see what his best effort could produce, given his available time, sedentary lifestyle, and degree of obesity. He gained the positive mind-set of "doing what it takes" to manage this for life.

For his program, Michael used meal replacements for breakfast and lunch, with raw vegetables as a between-meal snack. It was easy and convenient, and the unlimited veggies were a plus to balance the meal replacement shake or bar. The crunch of the vegetables also was a good stress reliever for him. Michael could adjust his schedule to be home from work between six and seven, and finish any remaining work in the evening, if needed. The couple ate together at a regular dinner time, and Nikki served portion-controlled dinners. Michael enjoyed an evening snack, and started an evening ritual of a glass of skim milk and his choice of a 100-calorie packaged snack, followed immediately by brushing his teeth, which signaled the end of the eating day.

It was hard for Michael to admit that it was tiring for him to increase his activity, due to his weight. He had no time for the gym, but agreed to wear a pedometer, and walk for five minutes at a time, six times a day, and add a twenty-minute walk with Nikki three times during the week, and on both weekend days. Nikki was his perfect exercise buddy, as she was supportive, stopped when Michael needed to pause when he got fatigued, and helped him meet his daily goals.

Michael was committed to a healthy lifestyle and lost 35 pounds in six months. While that is very positive weight-loss success, Michael spent a lot of time thinking about his ability to sustain this effort with lifestyle alone and his ability to lose another 100 pounds. After long discussions with Nikki, Michael felt he needed to add a power tool to sustain his effort and enthusiasm. He was evaluated for obesity surgery, with the support of his primary care doctor. After the appropriate medical, nutritional, and psychological screenings at a Center of Excellence facility, Michael's surgeon performed a gastric bypass.

Nine months after surgery, Michael had lost 75 more pounds. At twelve months, he had lost a total of 110 pounds. His total (including the first 35 pounds) weight loss was 145, which he has maintained for the past five years. He is vigilant with his mandatory dietary regimen, and takes vitamins and minerals daily. Nikki still helps him monitor adequate protein and fluid needs. He is walking forty minutes daily, and bought a treadmill to ensure his regular activity. He follows up yearly with his surgeon and primary care doctor, where he goes for bloodwork to monitor his nutritional needs. While Michael agrees that this lifestyle is tougher than any diet plan he had ever done, it was worth all the effort, and surgery was the key addition to his BEAM Box to support his long-term lifestyle success.

---

## Lifestyle Tools after Surgery: A Permanent Commitment

While a Center of Excellence–certified surgeon can provide you with a perfect operation and anatomical support, it is totally up to *you* to have a successful surgical outcome. By that I mean a *permanent commitment* to a lifestyle with restricted food intake. In our toxic eating environment, we are surrounded by food and temptation all the time, and we need to develop ways to avoid overindulging. The effort must be *unrelenting*. You can't go back to your old eating habits without bad physical consequences — vomiting, diarrhea, dehydration, just to name a few.

The main bonus of obesity surgery is that it really can make the lifestyle effort easier — but never easy! If you recognize that, you're already a step ahead.

**Lifestyle Basics after Surgery**

- Keep fluid intake up (6 to 8 glasses a day)
- Eat adequate protein (50 to 70 grams a day)
- Eat three to four small meals a day (no meal skipping)
- Take vitamins and minerals daily
- Walk a minimum of 30 minutes daily
- Learn to manage stress
- Ensure regular medical/surgical follow-up

While gastric banding and gastric bypass surgery are very different operations, the lifestyle part of the equation for long-term weight management remains the same. After surgery, you'll be given a specific eating plan for the early weeks after surgery. You'll progress from clear liquids (as with any other major surgery) to full liquids, to pureed foods, to a soft diet, and then to regular food. Vitamin and mineral supplementation, for life, is a given. While many people take only a multivitamin, others, particularly the gastric bypass group, need additional supplementation, including vitamin B12, iron, and calcium. For gastric banding, it takes about six weeks to reach a regular diet. For the gastric bypass, it takes about sixteen weeks to achieve it. You'll meet regularly with your surgeon during these early weeks to determine the right pace of diet advancement and to determine your own vitamin/mineral needs.

**Diet Phases after Surgery**

*Phase 1*: Clear Liquids (you can see through them)

Water, low-calorie juices, low-calorie sports drinks, beef/chicken/vegetable broth, decaf coffee, sugar-free popsicles

*Phase 2*: Full Liquids (includes clear liquids)
Skim milk, protein shakes, sugar-free nonfat yogurt, low-fat cream soups

*Phase 3*: Pureed Foods
Cottage cheese, scrambled eggs or egg substitute, baby foods, plain white fish varieties

*Phase 4*: Soft/Adaptive Foods

> Tuna fish, mashed potatoes, oatmeal, cooked vegetables, chopped white meat turkey/chicken breast, peeled fresh fruit

*Phase 5*: Stabilization (Regular Diet)

> Small amounts of nutrient-rich foods

Once you're at the stabilization, or regular diet, phase, you can utilize the food tools found in chapter 3. Remember, when you've healed from the anatomical adjustment of your digestive tract—which is what obesity surgery is—you'll have this power tool to help keep your calorie intake lower for the long term.

One word of caution: it is very easy to "eat around the surgery." If you want to consume extra calories, you can do so with high-calorie liquids. The surgery isn't foolproof. You've got to work hard to both lose the weight and keep it off. That's why a comprehensive lifestyle approach *after* the surgery is a key part of success.

Support is another strong part of success after obesity surgery. Staying on track with your new eating pattern, vitamin and mineral supplementation, and changing physical activity habits is hard, and we all need support at some point. If this sounds to you amazingly similar to nonsurgical weight loss, you're right. The surgical tool is one that makes the other tools easier to stick with—it does not replace them. With the surgery, you're really leveling the playing field and taking the opportunity to use these tools in a comprehensive way to make the lifestyle easier, whereas before the surgery, sustained weight loss continued to fail.

If you've included the power tool of bariatric surgery in your BEAM Box, you're now better equipped to adapt the lifestyle tools of eating, activity, and behavioral adjustments for both successful weight loss and long-term weight maintenance.

# 9

# Life after Weight Loss
## Body Contouring

It's a question on the minds of most people, but one that many are afraid or embarrassed to ask. What about body-contouring surgery after weight loss? All that effort to lose weight, and somehow our bodies don't just snap back into the mental image we had. For many, there's a lot of loose skin that even the most robust exercise cannot cure. Considering body contouring is a natural part of the weight-loss cycle and goes along with what I call looking good inside and out. While we are still the same person inside after weight loss, that extra skin hanging in all the wrong places can interfere with our quality of life. Plastic surgery to trim excess skin is not for everyone, but it's most certainly not an issue of vanity. Whether you've lost several hundred pounds or just a few, the decision to have the surgery, which can be an important tool in your BEAM Box, is a very personal one. Some people have a physical need to alleviate chafed skin and infections. Others seek a boost in self-esteem and quality of life. I'd like to discuss the pros and cons of body contouring after weight loss, and provide some guidelines on how to determine if it's right for you.

# Body-Contouring Basics

The surgical removal of extra hanging skin is the foundation of body contouring. Make no mistake. Body contouring is major surgery, with general anesthesia and everything else that surgery involves. When a patient asks what body-contouring procedures he or she needs, my favorite response is, "*Nothing.*" You don't *need* anything, but a discussion of what you might *want* to improve your quality of life is a must-do.

I'd like to separate myth from fact when it comes to body-contouring surgery, liposuction, and cosmetic fillers after weight loss. An informed decision can be made, once you have the facts. Body contouring is not right for everyone, and only you can decide if it can be a useful tool for you.

## What Is Body-Contouring Surgery?

Body-contouring surgery removes the excess hanging skin from virtually any part of the body, including the face and neck, thighs, buttocks, arms, breasts, stomach, and chest or upper body.

I'm often asked if I think someone has "enough extra skin to remove." My answer is always the same: the extra skin is only a problem if it bothers you. It's important to figure out what parts of your body you'd like to modify. You might immediately reply, "Everything." Not so fast. Think about what you're looking for. Do you want a more youthful face, and to get rid of your "turkey neck"? Does your belly skin bother you? Do your thighs applaud when you walk? Do you avoid wearing sleeveless clothing because your arms bother you? While all of these topics will come up when you meet with your plastic surgeon, it's a good idea to think about your particular problem areas beforehand.

Procedures vary for each body part, and you'll want to discuss the specifics of each with your surgeon. This kind of surgery can involve more than just removing extra skin; it usually includes tightening of underlying muscle groups, and sometimes using implants, particularly for the breasts.

Sometimes multiple body parts are done as a single procedure, called a "total body lift," which involves the thighs, buttocks, and abdominal area. Liposuction (removal of fat tissue using a vacuum-like approach) is often added to refine the surgical procedures.

## How to Use Body Contouring as a Weight-Management Tool

Don't make the mistake of thinking body contouring is a replacement for weight loss. Some people think of body contouring as simply cutting off extra fat and actually replacing a weight-loss effort. Body contouring is most effective when people are pretty close to their target weight. It's a matter of removing the extra skin (which can weigh as little as 3 pounds to as much as 30) in a surgical procedure. It's considered major surgery, and you can expect a hospital stay of up to one day.

Liposuction is often combined with surgery to *refine* the surgical procedure but not to replace it. Liposuction, when used alone, can produce a contoured look, but it is effective for only smaller areas of excess skin. (On the horizon is a kind of liposuction said to remove several dozen pounds of extra fat; this is experimental right now but may be available in the future for general use.) As with body-contouring surgery, don't make the mistake of thinking that liposuction is a mode of weight loss— somehow vacuuming your excess pounds away. It's simply a tool to refine a body size pretty close to a target weight.

What do I mean by a target? I *don't* mean a weight that matches the standardized charts, of a body mass index lower than 25. I mean a weight at which your health is improved, and that you can maintain with moderate, not heroic, effort. The goal of body contouring is improved appearance, and sometimes physical health.

For some, the hanging skin presents a hygiene problem—causing recurrent infections and skin irritation from rubbing against other body parts. A commonly reported skin irritation occurs when walking, due to thigh skin rubbing together. This can interfere with daily walking, running, or other physical activity. Other problems include rashes from hanging belly skin.

An important thing to remember when using body contouring in your BEAM Box is that the newly tightened skin helps serve as a permanent reminder to avoid weight regain. If you gain weight, this skin doesn't really stretch much, and you'll feel a tightness that will remind you to get back on the lifestyle track. While that might sound scary, it's a big help for many people and a real sign that you're dedicated to lifelong weight management.

Another thing to remember is that while liposuction *permanently* removes the fat cells that have been suctioned out, all the fat cells remaining in other body parts are perfectly able to fill up with additional fat if you regain some weight. This is another good deterrent to weight regain, since you'll find the extra pounds can pop up in other places, giving you a lumpy look, the opposite of what was gained by the original procedure.

## When to Consider Body Contouring

You'll want to think about body contouring *at the end* of active weight loss. It's most effective as one of your maintenance tools. Your lifestyle is an integral part of long-term success—a healthy diet supports good wound healing of the scar line. (Yes, there are scars, but they fade with time.) A protein-dense diet and a variety of fruits and vegetables provide both the extra protein and the mix of vitamins and minerals needed to support wound healing. It's also a good idea to take a daily multivitamin/mineral supplement for nutritional insurance. If you smoke, you'll have to quit, which will be good for you for a lot of reasons but is a must-do for body-contouring surgery. Many surgeons will not perform the surgery if you're a smoker.

You need to think long and hard about what you expect from body-contouring surgery. Realistic expectations are essential to a happy outcome. It's important to discuss this with your surgeon, and ask specific questions about your own body. It's not only about how you'll look, but how your life will be affected. If you were a happy person before, you'll be a happy person afterward. If you have problems in your relationships, body contouring isn't going to fix them. Job woes won't get any better, and you won't get promoted if your skin is tighter.

I recall the surprise of one patient who, after weight loss and a tummy tuck (abdominoplasty), was amazed that she had been stood up by a date. "I looked so good and had such a flat stomach," she recalled. While this might seem exaggerated to you, the take-home message is to consider body contouring as an improvement to your quality of life. Do sagging arms really make a difference to you? One woman wanted to get her arms done only because her young children kept swatting them, to see them flap around, finding it amusing. This young mother, Christine, was motivated to put a stop to this, and did. You can read her story on page 206.

It's not a matter of vanity. If this tool appeals to you, read on to learn how to find a plastic surgeon who is a good match for you.

### Barbara's Story
## My Hanging Skin Is an Alien!

Barbara, age forty-two, is a long-term weight-loss success story. After working hard on her BEAM Box, Barbara had lost 75 pounds in a year and a half and had kept it off for four years. She had taken a long and honest look at her barriers and worked hard to find solutions to the sabotages that had interfered with past weight-loss efforts. Sounds good, right? Barbara came to see me with a feeling of sadness she had finally figured out. While she was thrilled with her weight loss, she had a lot of hanging skin that bothered her. "I'm not vain," she said. She felt great, and agreed that good health was its own reward. So what was the matter? Barbara confessed that her extra belly skin felt "like an alien" that she tucked into her pants every day. "It doesn't even feel like it belongs to me," she said. Hiding the skin was easy, under clothes or with uncomfortable body slimmers, but she always knew it was there, and she felt worse about it month after month. Barbara came to see me feeling very guilty about wanting to do some-thing about her extra skin. She thought that if she did so, she was just being shallow and self-indulgent. "I should be happy and content with my weight loss, but I'm not," she said glumly. "My boyfriend doesn't mind, so why should I?"

Barbara visited a plastic surgeon specializing in body contouring to learn what could be done to help her. He praised her for maintaining her weight loss, which is essential to a long-term successful visual outcome. Barbara had an abdominoplasty, which involved removing the loose skin from her abdomen and also tightening the abdominal muscles. After wearing a "binder" (girdle) for a few weeks during the healing process, Barbara was thrilled with her result. She was surprised at what a difference she felt, and was delighted every day when she put on her jeans and could skip the "tuck." Her boyfriend still loved her just the same, tuck or no tuck, but Barbara knew that she had done it as an expression of love for herself. It was an important, final addition to her BEAM Box.

## How to Find the Best Surgeon for You

While you might think the decision to go ahead with body-contouring surgery is the hardest, finding the right surgeon for you is equally important. Word-of-mouth referrals—from a trusted friend or relative—are often a good place to start. Once you have that name, you must still do your homework.

Here are important criteria for choosing a plastic surgeon. Whether you had a personal referral or found a surgeon from an online resource, ask these six questions when you call the office for the first time. Flashy ads and wild promises don't tell the whole story (usually not even part of it). While many physicians advertise plastic surgery services, it's important to make sure you have a qualified professional *in plastic surgery.* You must complete this step before including body contouring in this part of the BEAM Box. Consider the following important questions:

1. **Is he or she board certified in plastic surgery?** Ideally, you'll want a surgeon who is board certified from the American College of Plastic

and Reconstructive Surgery. (Note: Some ophthalmologists, who are board certified from the American College of Ophthalmology, have specialized training and have extended the scope of practice to cosmetic eye surgery, in additional to general eye surgery. If you seek only localized eye procedures, you may want to explore that option. Similarly, some board-certified head and neck surgeons have additional training in some cosmetic procedures. Ask about your doctor's specific training and certifications in your particular area of body-contouring interest.)

2. **Does he or she operate in a hospital (not office) setting?** You'll want to make sure procedures are done in a hospital, with major medical backup if there is an emergency. While "surgi-centers" abound, if you are the person with a surprising complication, you'll want to be in a major hospital with immediate medical attention. While some small procedures, including liposuction, are done in the office, most are done in the hospital. These might be "day procedures"—no overnight stay—but you have the comfort and security of a hospital setting. There is a lot of variability in the surgi-center approach. Only a discussion with your surgeon can help you decide if this venue is appropriate for you.

3. **Does he or she specialize in your particular type of surgery?** It is the rare plastic surgeon who specializes in the "whole body," so ask about the personal body parts you're interested in. Ask how many of your particular procedures are done yearly. Who is part of the surgical team? If you're at an academic medical center that is also a teaching hospital (for residents), ask how much of your procedure is done by your surgeon. (The right answer: all of it!)

4. **Can you see some patient photos for your specific procedure?** When it comes to body-contouring surgery, a picture's worth a thousand words. Your surgeon should have photos to show you of a typical outcome—no matter what body part you're interested in. You'll want to ask to see before-and-after photos of someone whose starting point was similar to your own.

5. **What type of follow-up can you expect?** You'll want a complete description of your postoperative process. It should be organized, and include emergency contacts and a specific plan of follow-up visits. Ask about both short-term and long-term follow-up. Do you have a list of numbers and resources to guide you? You should feel comfortable that there is a whole team to help support both your preoperative and postoperative experience. Important questions include when to call the doctor, how much swelling is normal, how long the swelling lasts, and any special garments you'll need to wear afterward (oftentimes a "compression" shirt or shorts are recommended for several weeks).

6. **What is his or her personal complication rate?** While some people feel it is insulting to ask about complication rate, that information is essential. You'll want some answers to not only how often complications occur with your particular surgeon (don't settle for general numbers), but also how they're handled, and any long-term implications this could have for you.

At the end of this discussion, you should feel confident that you and your surgeon are a good match. Do your homework in this area in order to make surgery a safe and effective tool. You'll be glad you did. One final thought: while you can accumulate this information on your own, there are plastic surgery consultants who can help you sort through the dozens of plastic surgeons you might consider in your area. It will be a separate fee, but it might be worth the cost for the added peace of mind.

### Christine's Success Story
## My "Hanging" Arms

Christine was a thirty-eight-year-old mother of two girls, ages three and five, who had worked hard to lose 50 pounds she'd accumulated over the past twenty years. Her BEAM Box was complete and only needed minor tool adjustments from time to time. As a dental hygienist who worked part-time, Christine felt she had an excellent balance between her professional and her family activities. During the summer, the family spent most of their free time in their backyard pool.

Christine's eyes welled up with tears as she explained to me that her younger daughter loved to play with her hanging arm skin. It was an innocent and loving activity, which Christine understood, and they all had a good laugh when her daughter described it as "Play-Doh." Privately, Christine was terribly upset and couldn't stop thinking about it. While she had worked hard at toning her muscles, she agreed that she had a lot of extra surrounding skin that no amount of exercise could shrink. After a visit with a plastic surgeon, Christine was pleased to see that she could have just her arm skin removed in a procedure called a brachioplasty. Christine could not have been more pleased with the result. With the extra skin removed, her toned arms looked strong and sleek. Her months of weight lifting had defined her muscles, which had been hidden under the hanging skin. The surgery was a final added tool for Christine's BEAM Box, which provided a big lift to her positive body image.

---

## Will Insurance Pay for It?

A loaded question in the realm of plastic surgery is always, who pays? In a perfect world, body contouring would be a covered service, but most often it's not. Some procedures, usually for hanging belly skin (called a "panniculectomy," after the "pannus," which is that fatty apron that hangs down over the lower abdomen), are covered by some insurance plans. Usually the condition must be considered a medical condition (skin irritation, infections, and chafing) and not a cosmetic issue. Many plans will require documentation of these medical conditions by a dermatologist or primary care physician. This coverage area is truly gray. When meeting with your surgeon, ask about insurance coverage, but don't expect much.

When it comes to body contouring, for many people, where there's a will, there's a way. Saving money, taking a loan, or adjusting the number or type of procedures are all possibilities. There is usually a staff member in the surgeon's office to discuss the financials with you. This type of surgery can be affordable, and there are actually published and recommended fees for each procedure from the American Academy of Plastic and Reconstructive Surgery. And don't be shy. Discuss your concerns with your surgeon, to determine the best plan for both your body and your wallet.

## Nonsurgical Options: All about Fillers

A final word about what's sometimes called "nonsurgical" body contouring, referring to the face. These are injections of what's commonly known as "fillers"—Food and Drug Administration–approved compounds injected into facial areas to "plump up" sagging areas and reduce lines and creases. Taking your own body fat from other areas of the body, such as the buttocks, is also an option. There are a variety of these compounds, based on their different "bead" size, for use in fine lines (along the chin) or deeper folds (between the nose and mouth). Another popular option for lines in the upper face, eyes, and forehead is Botox, the popular botulinum toxin that temporarily paralyzes the muscles of the injected area. Both types of compounds have side effects, and the risk-to-benefit ratio might not be worth it to you. These treatments are temporary (the effects last three to six months, roughly), and can be somewhat painful. While topical anesthetics are applied to the face, needles are still used for injections. Here are the most common used fillers.

| Popular Name | Chemical Compound |
| --- | --- |
| Restylane, Juvederm, Perlane | Hyaluronic acid |
| Zyplast, Cosmoderm, Artecoll | Collagen |
| Evolence | Collagen matrix |
| Sculptra | Poly-L-lactic acid |
| Radiesse, Radiance | Calcium-based microspheres in water-based gel |
| Artefill | PMMA non-absorbable microspheres |

These might be an option for you if facial lines and wrinkles are an issue and you are willing to pay for this regularly. It's a matter of quality of life—if you feel better having those lines and wrinkles smoothed out, it's a great thing. You should feel happy and empowered that these tools are available. As with all medical procedures of this type, you'll want to make sure yours is done by a board-certified plastic surgeon or a board-certified dermatologist.

And as with all medical and surgical procedures, an open and honest talk with your doctor will provide realistic expectations and a full understanding of the risks and benefits of body contouring—whether you seek permanent major adjustments (as with surgical body contouring and liposuction) or temporary solutions to your appearance (with fillers).

# The Real You Recipe File

Here are some of my favorite recipes. They are mostly single-serving size (or sometimes serve two or three when indicated), but they can be easily doubled, tripled, or more, depending on how many people you are cooking for. Cooking for one? Just divide up the servings for another meal. Refrigerate for up to three days, or freeze for a later meal.

## Breakfast

### Bagel 'n Lox

- 1 scooped regular, 100-calorie, or Weight Watchers bagel
- 1 tablespoon reduced-fat cream cheese
- 3 ounces Nova smoked salmon (lox)
- 2 slices red onion
- 2 slices tomato
- Capers (optional)
- 2 leaves of romaine or other lettuce

If using a regular full-size bagel, scoop out most of the doughy inside; or use a Weight Watchers bagel, or a 100-calorie regular bagel. Slice in half, and toast if desired. Spread the cream cheese on both halves, and top each half with smoked salmon, a slice of red onion, and a slice of tomato. Add capers if desired. Top each half with lettuce leaf.

## Easy Vegetable Frittata

2 whole eggs, or 1 egg and 5 whites, or ½ cup liquid egg substitute
¼ cup each chopped onions, peppers, and mushrooms
Oil spray

Beat the egg mixture until light and frothy. Set stove to medium heat. Spray a nonstick pan with oil spray and place it on the burner. Add the egg mixture and swirl in the pan. Allow eggs to set until cooked around the edges. Scatter the vegetables over the top of the egg mixture, and cook until eggs are set (about 3 minutes). Using a spatula, fold the frittata in half, and gently slide onto a plate.

## Fruit and Nut Oatmeal

Single-serve pack of plain instant oatmeal
1 tablespoon chopped walnuts
1 tablespoon dried cranberries
¼ cup skim milk

Prepare oatmeal as directed on the package. Let stand for 2 minutes to thicken, and add ¼ cup skim milk (heated in microwave, if desired, for 10 seconds on high). Sprinkle with dried cranberries and chopped nuts.

## PB and J Waffle

1 Kashi, Eggo, Van's, or other whole grain waffle
1 teaspoon peanut butter (smooth or crunchy)
4 sliced strawberries

Toast the waffle as directed. Spread the peanut butter to cover the waffle. Add the sliced strawberries.

## Quick and Tasty Egg Sandwich

2 eggs, or 5 egg whites and 1 whole egg, or ½ cup liquid egg substitute
1 slice 2% cheddar cheese
1 100-calorie 100% whole wheat English muffin
Hot sauce (optional)

In a small bowl, beat the whole eggs or egg mixture of choice. You can cook the eggs in a nonstick pan, but here's an even quicker and mess-free option. Put the eggs into a paper cup and cover with a paper towel. Cook in the microwave on high for 30 seconds, and stir. Cook for another 15 seconds, until eggs are cooked through and not runny. Cut the English muffin in half and toast it. Take one-half of the muffin and put the slice of cheese on top. Microwave for 15 seconds, or until melted. Remove from microwave and add cooked eggs. Top with the remaining muffin half. Serve with hot sauce, if desired.

## Tomato and Cheese Omelet

2 whole eggs, or 5 egg whites and 1 whole egg, or ½ cup egg substitute
3 tablespoons skim milk or soy milk
¼ cup shredded 2% cheddar cheese
1 chopped fresh Roma tomato or 4 ounces chopped canned tomatoes

In a small bowl, beat the whole eggs, or egg mixture of choice, with 3 tablespoons of skim milk (or soy milk if preferred). Spray a 6-inch nonstick skillet with a vegetable oil spray and set the pan on medium heat for 1 minute. Add the egg mixture and spread in pan. Cook until edges are firm and set. Sprinkle the cheese across the top and add the chopped tomatoes. As cheese begins to melt, fold omelet in half and continue cooking until bottom is brown. Using a spatula, flip the omelet and cook until the other side is brown, about 1 minute.

## Yogurt Parfait

8 ounces sugar-free nonfat regular or Greek-style yogurt
1 cup frozen or fresh blueberries
¼ cup crushed Special K Protein Plus cereal or Fiber One Clusters cereal
Maraschino cherries (optional)

Place half the yogurt at the bottom of a tall glass. Top with half the berries and half the crushed cereal. Repeat with remaining ingredients. Add one or two maraschino cherries on top for an added treat (optional).

# Lunch

## Bean Burrito

1 small whole wheat tortilla
½ cup canned fat-free refried beans
½ cup shredded 2% cheddar cheese
¼ cup mild or medium salsa (fresh or jarred)

Spread tortilla with refried beans and sprinkle with shredded cheese. Microwave on high for 30 seconds. Remove to plate, top with salsa, and roll up.

## Buffalo Chicken Fingers

4 ounces chicken tenders (about four strips)
1 beaten egg white
Panko (or regular) bread crumbs
Sriracha sauce

Dip each chicken tender in the egg white and coat lightly in bread crumbs. Place on a cookie sheet coated with olive oil spray. Spray chicken tenders lightly before baking in preheated 375 degree oven for 8 minutes. Turn over, spray again, and bake an additional 8 minutes, until crispy. Serve with sriracha sauce.

## Chicken Caesar Salad

4 cups romaine (washed and dried)
1 skinless, cooked chicken breast (about 5 ounces)
¼ cup shredded Parmesan cheese
¼ cup large-cut prepared croutons
3 tablespoons fat-free Caesar dressing

Tear romaine into bite-sized pieces. Cut the chicken into pieces and add to the romaine. Add the Parmesan cheese and croutons, and toss with dressing.

## Lettuce Wraps

4 large romaine lettuce leaves
4 ounces cooked sliced white meat chicken (deli, roasted prepackaged, or leftover rotisserie breast meat)
1 cup shredded carrots
1 cup fresh bean sprouts
1 cup chopped celery
Ken's Asian Salad Dressing Spray

Spread each lettuce leaf with one-quarter of the chicken and each vegetable. Spray each leaf 6 times with dressing, distributing over the whole surface. Roll tightly, starting from the large leafy end.

## My Favorite Vegetable Soup (An Anytime Food)

*Serving size: 1 cup*
10 cups low-sodium beef broth (use water if preferred)
1 large can (28 ounces) chopped tomatoes in thick puree
2 medium onions, chopped

4 each: large carrots, parsnips, and celery stalks, all cut into ½-inch chunks

1 pound fresh or frozen green beans, cut in 1-inch pieces

1 small head cabbage, coarsely chopped

Pour beef broth (or water) into a large stock pot along with canned tomatoes and puree. Add onions, carrots, parsnips, celery. Bring to a boil, then reduce to a simmer. Cover and cook for 20 minutes. Add green beans and cabbage and return to a boil. Turn down the heat to a gentle simmer and cook for an additional 20 minutes. This recipe makes a lot of soup, so I like to freeze half for later and keep the rest ready to eat in the fridge.

## Taco Salad

3 cups mixed greens

⅔ cup low-fat chili (purchased or homemade, lean-beef or bean)

¼ cup shredded 2% cheese

10 baked tortilla chips (optional)

Place greens on a large plate. Top with chili of your choice (a small Wendy's chili makes this recipe easy). Make sure the chili is hot so the cheese melts when you sprinkle it on top. Serve with baked tortilla chips. (If you want to go chip-free, you'll have an additional 100 calories to spend on an extra snack.)

## Tuna-Spinach Wrap

3-ounce can chunk light tuna packed in water

½ ounce 2% shredded cheddar cheese

Chopped onions, peppers, cucumbers, tomatoes

4 cups raw spinach (washed and dried)

3 tablespoons fat-free Italian dressing

Light whole grain flat bread wrap (90 to 100 calories)

Place the raw spinach in a bowl. Drain the tuna and flake it with a fork while adding to the spinach. Add chopped vegetables and shredded cheese. Mix with dressing. Spread the mixture on the wrap and roll it up.

## Tuna Tortilla

3-ounce can light tuna, water packed

1 tablespoon light mayonnaise

1 6-inch whole wheat tortilla

1 medium stalk celery, chopped

2 lettuce leaves (your choice), shredded or finely chopped

Drain the tuna and place it in a small bowl. Mix in light mayonnaise and celery until well blended, mashing together with a fork. Spread the tuna salad on the tortilla, top it with shredded lettuce, and roll it up.

## Twist on a Cobb Salad

3 cups romaine lettuce, washed and dried

¼ cup chopped turkey or chicken breast pieces

¼ cup chopped lean deli ham

1 ounce shredded reduced-fat cheese

2 chopped hard-boiled egg whites

2 tablespoons prepared guacamole

6 grape tomatoes

6 black olives

2 tablespoons fat-free vinaigrette dressing

Tear romaine into bite-sized pieces and place on a flat plate. Make a "composed" salad with the rest of the ingredients by placing them side-by-side on top of the greens. Arrange a column of turkey or chicken, then ham, then cheese, then egg whites, then guacamole. Sprinkle top of salad with grape tomatoes and black olives. Drizzle fat-free vinaigrette over the top.

## Quick Chicken BLT Wrap

1 light whole wheat wrap, plain or Italian-flavored

4 ounces cooked and diced white meat chicken (deli, roasted prepackaged, leftover rotisserie breast meat)

5 grape tomatoes, cut into quarters

1 tablespoon Bac-Os or Real Bacon Bits

½ cup shredded lettuce

1 teaspoon light mayonnaise

Spread the wrap with light mayonnaise. Add the diced chicken, and top with tomatoes, bacon bits, and lettuce. Tuck in the sides, and roll tightly.

# Dinner

## Baked Salmon and Asparagus

16-ounce salmon fillet

4 stalks asparagus, cut into 2-inch pieces

Dried tarragon, black pepper to taste

½ cup dry vermouth or other white wine

Preheat oven to 350 degrees. Place salmon in a baking dish, season with black pepper, and sprinkle with dried tarragon. Add asparagus pieces around the salmon. Pour ½ cup wine into the dish and bake uncovered (middle rack) until liquid starts to bubble. Baste the salmon with the liquid every 5 minutes, for a total cooking time of about 12 minutes, until the salmon feels springy to the touch and is cooked through. For a drier fillet, cook a total of 15 minutes.

## Beef-Vegetable Kabobs

*Serves 2*

10 ounces beef top round, cut into 8 pieces

1 whole green or red sweet pepper, cut into 8 pieces

1 large red onion, cut into 8 pieces

8 cherry tomatoes

½ cup low-calorie bottled Italian dressing

Place beef pieces in a flat glass dish with sides (a 9 ×12 Pyrex dish or glass pie plate, for example) and pierce in several places with a fork. Pour Italian dressing over meat and marinate in the refrigerator for at least 45 minutes, but not more than 4 hours. Mix occasionally. Spray 2 large skewers with nonstick spray, and alternate meat and vegetables to make two kabobs. Before preheating the grill (outside or oven), spray grids with Pam High Heat cooking spray to avoid sticking. Grill 3 inches from heat, for about 10 minutes, and turn. Cook for an additional 10 minutes (for medium doneness).

## Crustless Peach Pie

1 large peach, sliced (or 1 cup frozen peach slices, or water-packed canned peaches)

1 teaspoon brown sugar

¼ teaspoon cinnamon

Place peaches in a microwave-safe shallow bowl. Mix brown sugar and cinnamon together, and sprinkle evenly over the peaches. Cover, and microwave on high for 1 minute (up to 2 minutes if using fresh peaches).

## Cucumber and Onion Salad

*Serves 2*

1 large cucumber, peeled and sliced thinly

½ medium red onion, sliced thinly

⅛ cup rice wine vinegar

⅛ cup Splenda

Place cucumber and onion in a large bowl. Mix rice wine vinegar together with Splenda. Toss with cucumber/onion mix. While this can be served immediately, it's even better when allowed to marinate for 1 to 2 hours before serving.

## Deluxe Veggie Burger

1 Flame-Grilled Boca Burger

1 slice 2% cheddar cheese or soy cheese

Leaf of romaine lettuce

Sliced tomato and onion

2 teaspoons prepared honey mustard

1 "light" whole wheat sandwich bun

Cook burger according to directions, in microwave or pan. Add cheese, and microwave for 15 seconds until melted. Place burger on bun and spread with honey mustard, adding tomato, onion, and lettuce before topping with remaining half of bun.

## Easy Teriyaki Pork Tenderloin

*Serves 3*

1 pound fresh pork tenderloin (or teriyaki premarinated package)

½ cup prepared teriyaki sauce

Preheat oven to 350 degrees. If using premarinated tenderloin, open package and transfer the tenderloin to a baking dish, making sure to include package marinade in the cooking pan. If using a fresh tenderloin, place it in a glass dish, prick meat with a fork, and cover with teriyaki sauce. Cover and marinate in the refrigerator for 1 to 3 hours. Cook tenderloin for about 30 minutes, or until an instant thermometer registers 165 degrees.

## Hearty Meat Sauce

*Serves 3*

8 ounces cooked extra-lean beef (92% fat-free or higher) or ready-to-use browned soy crumbles

1 large can (28 ounces) chopped tomatoes in thick tomato puree

1 small can (4 ounces) tomato paste

2 cloves fresh garlic, minced (or equivalent jarred in water)

1 tablespoon dried mixed Italian seasonings

Spray a nonstick skillet with oil spray, and brown chopped beef over medium high heat (or start with precooked soy crumbles). Add tomatoes and tomato paste, chopped garlic, and Italian seasonings. Simmer covered for 40 minutes. Correct seasonings. Serve over whole wheat or flax pasta.

## Hearty Mushroom Barley Soup

*Serving size: 1½ cups*

1 large onion, chopped

3 large carrots, chopped

3 large celery stalks, chopped

2 teaspoons minced garlic jarred in water, or 4 fresh garlic cloves

2 pounds mushrooms, sliced

½ teaspoon ground pepper, additional to taste

1 cup raw pearl barley, rinsed

3 quarts low-sodium beef broth

1 quart water

Spray a large stock pot or large kettle with vegetable spray, and add onion, celery, carrots, and garlic. Cook over medium heat for 3 minutes, until softened. Add all remaining ingredients, bring to a boil, then turn down the heat and simmer gently for about 2 hours until barley is tender. Stir occasionally (about every 20 minutes). Add additional pepper if desired. (Note: When reheating, the barley continues to swell and thicken the soup, and you may need to add additional hot water to thin to desired consistency.)

## Marinated Grilled Flank Steak

*Serves 3*

1 pound whole flank steak

½ cup reduced-fat Italian dressing

Using the prongs of a fork, prick holes in raw flank steak on both sides. Coat with salad dressing, and marinate in a covered dish for 1 to 4 hours in the refrigerator. Preheat grill to medium-high for 20 minutes (or put oven on broil). Cook steak for 8 minutes before turning. Cook another 5 to 8 minutes, or until an instant meat thermometer registers 165 degrees. Let meat rest for 5 minutes before slicing. Serving size is 3 to 4 slices, or about ⅓ of the total cooked meat.

## One-Minute Baked Apple

1 medium crisp apple (Fuji, Granny Smith, Rome, Gala, or similar)
1 teaspoon sugar or low-calorie sugar substitute
½ teaspoon cinnamon

Cut apple into quarters and remove seeds and core. Mix sugar and cinnamon is small bowl. Place apples on a microwave-safe plate and sprinkle with sugar and cinnamon. Microwave on high for 2 minutes, or until soft.

## Oven-Baked Garlic Fries

1 medium white potato
½ teaspoon paprika
½ teaspoon garlic powder
1 teaspoon olive oil
Pinch of salt

Preheat oven to 375 degrees. Cut potato, leaving skin on, into six wedges and toss with olive oil. In a separate dish, mix paprika, garlic powder, and salt. Rub the wedges with the seasoning mix and roast for 35 minutes or until crisp.

## Quick and Easy Stir-Fry

*Serves 2*
½ pound fresh chicken tenders
1 pound bag frozen vegetables (your choice: broccoli-cauliflower mix or a stir-fry blend go well here)

1 can sliced water chestnuts

½ cup prepared stir-fry cooking sauce, any variety (reduced sodium, if available)

1 cup shredded fresh Chinese (Napa) cabbage (optional)

Cut chicken tenders into 1-inch pieces. Microwave frozen vegetables for half the time listed on the package. In a large nonstick skillet coated with vegetable spray, sauté chicken for 2 minutes, or until white and opaque; remove and set aside. Place partly cooked vegetables in the pan, add stir-fry sauce, and cook for 2 minutes. Add chicken and water chestnuts, combine thoroughly, and cook for an additional 2 minutes. Top with shredded Chinese cabbage if desired before serving.

## Roasted Green Beans

½ pound fresh green beans, washed and dried

1 teaspoon olive oil (dark green, first press)

½ teaspoon kosher or sea salt (optional)

½ teaspoon ground black pepper

Spray a shallow pan with olive oil spray. Mix green beans with oil. Add pepper, and if desired, salt. Roast in preheated 450-degree oven for 12 to 15 minutes, to desired tenderness. Check beans after 10 minutes; if they seem dry, spray lightly with olive oil spray and roast for another few minutes until done.

## Savory Shrimp Scampi

5 large raw shrimp

1 tablespoon olive oil (dark green, first press)

Chopped fresh garlic (clove or jarred in water)

¼ of a fresh lemon

In a small nonstick skillet, heat the olive oil on medium-high until barely smoking. Add 1 fresh chopped garlic clove and cook for 1 to 2 minutes.

Add the raw shrimp and cook for 3 minutes, or until the shrimp have turned completely pink. Squirt a wedge of lemon across the shrimp and into the pan. Spoon shrimp and pan juices onto serving plate.

## Turkey Cacciatore

*Serves 4*

1 pound ground white meat turkey

1 large can (28 ounces) chopped tomatoes in tomato puree

1 large can (28 ounces) tomato sauce

1 small can (6 ounces) tomato paste

1 tablespoon dried oregano

1 tablespoon dried basil

1 tablespoon garlic powder

1 large onion, finely chopped

1 large green pepper, finely chopped

In a large nonstick skillet coated with vegetable spray, sauté the ground turkey until it is cooked through, making sure to separate into small pieces. Add the tomatoes, tomato sauce, tomato paste, spices, and chopped onion and pepper. Mix thoroughly, bring to a boil, and then reduce to a simmer for 30 minutes.

## White Beans and Greens with Polenta

*Serves 2*

1 cup cannellini (white pinto) beans

10 leaves of fresh escarole, torn in thirds

1 chopped medium onion

1 15-ounce can chopped tomatoes, with juice

½ small can (2 ounces) tomato paste

Instant polenta (cornmeal) or precooked polenta loaf

In a nonstick skillet, mix liquid from beans, canned tomatoes, tomato paste, and 2 ounces of hot water until smooth. Mix in chopped onion and beans. Place escarole pieces on top and cover tightly. Cook for 15 minutes at medium heat, until escarole is wilted. Serve in a shallow soup bowl. If desired, prepare instant polenta as directed, and place a 3-by-3 inch piece in the bowl as a base for the beans and greens. If using the polenta loaf, slice off 2 half-inch slices per serving.

# Understanding Your BMI

We all want to drop extra weight to look good, but it's also important to know if those extra pounds are putting your health at risk. That's where the body mass index (BMI) comes in. The BMI compares a person's height and weight, providing a single number that is a reasonable predictor of health risk related to extra weight. The BMI has replaced those charts of height and weight, and already accounts for frame size. Look at the chart on pages 228–229 and match up your current weight and height, and slide across to find your BMI. You can also calculate your own BMI by taking your weight (in pounds) and multiplying it by 703. Divide that number by your height (in inches), and take the resulting number and divide it by your height (in inches).

Once you know your BMI, you can honestly evaluate where you are on the health-risk scale of weight problems, not how you look in clothes. The higher your BMI, the higher your risk of weight-related illnesses. The goal of effective weight loss is to lose enough weight to resolve any medical issues, and not necessarily to fall into the "ideal" BMI range. The BMI risk chart is based on evidence-based population data, which cannot always apply to each of us as individuals.

| BMI | Classification | Disease Risk Waist Circumference (inches) | |
|---|---|---|---|
| | | Women (<35) Men (<40) | Women (35+) Men (40+) |
| Below 18.5 | Underweight | | |
| 18.5 – 24.9 | Healthy Weight | | |
| 25.0 – 29.9 | Overweight | Increased | High |
| 30.0 – 34.9 | Obesity – Class 1 | High | Very High |
| 35.0 – 39.9 | Obesity – Class 2 | Very High | Very High |
| 40 and above | Obesity – Class 3 | Extremely High | Extremely High |

Plus, where your weight is carried is a second predictor of health risk. The weight around your abdomen (belly fat) proves to be a greater health risk, even if the total amount of extra weight is not much. And for those of you in the overweight and moderately obese categories, losing just 5 to 10 percent of your starting weight can have a major impact on your health. For someone at 160 pounds, that's as little as 8 pounds.

Pay attention to your waist circumference. Studies clearly show that a larger waistline poses greater risk, even for those with a healthy BMI. Get out your tape measure and add this to your BMI result. Then, check out your numbers and your relative disease risk. This is your starting point from which to map your progress.

| Body Mass Index | | | | | | | | | | | | | | | | | |
|---|---|---|---|---|---|---|---|---|---|---|---|---|---|---|---|---|---|
| | Normal | | | | | | Overweight | | | | | Obese | | | | | |
| BMI | 19 | 20 | 21 | 22 | 23 | 24 | 25 | 26 | 27 | 28 | 29 | 30 | 31 | 32 | 33 | 34 | 35 | 36 |
| Height (inches) | Body Weight (pounds) | | | | | | | | | | | | | | | | |
| 58 | 91 | 96 | 100 | 105 | 110 | 115 | 119 | 124 | 129 | 134 | 138 | 143 | 148 | 153 | 158 | 162 | 167 | 172 |
| 59 | 94 | 99 | 104 | 109 | 114 | 119 | 124 | 128 | 133 | 138 | 143 | 148 | 153 | 158 | 163 | 168 | 173 | 178 |
| 60 | 97 | 102 | 107 | 112 | 118 | 123 | 128 | 133 | 138 | 143 | 148 | 153 | 158 | 163 | 168 | 174 | 179 | 184 |
| 61 | 100 | 106 | 111 | 116 | 122 | 127 | 132 | 137 | 143 | 148 | 153 | 158 | 164 | 169 | 174 | 180 | 185 | 190 |
| 62 | 104 | 109 | 115 | 120 | 126 | 131 | 136 | 142 | 147 | 153 | 158 | 164 | 169 | 175 | 180 | 186 | 191 | 196 |
| 63 | 107 | 113 | 118 | 124 | 130 | 135 | 141 | 146 | 152 | 158 | 163 | 169 | 175 | 180 | 186 | 191 | 197 | 203 |
| 64 | 110 | 116 | 122 | 128 | 134 | 140 | 145 | 151 | 157 | 163 | 169 | 174 | 180 | 186 | 192 | 197 | 204 | 209 |
| 65 | 114 | 120 | 126 | 132 | 138 | 144 | 150 | 156 | 162 | 168 | 174 | 180 | 186 | 192 | 198 | 204 | 210 | 216 |
| 66 | 118 | 124 | 130 | 136 | 142 | 148 | 155 | 161 | 167 | 173 | 179 | 186 | 192 | 198 | 204 | 210 | 216 | 223 |
| 67 | 121 | 127 | 134 | 140 | 146 | 153 | 159 | 166 | 172 | 178 | 185 | 191 | 198 | 204 | 211 | 217 | 223 | 230 |
| 68 | 125 | 131 | 138 | 144 | 151 | 158 | 164 | 171 | 177 | 184 | 190 | 197 | 203 | 210 | 216 | 223 | 230 | 236 |
| 69 | 128 | 135 | 142 | 149 | 155 | 162 | 169 | 176 | 182 | 189 | 196 | 203 | 209 | 216 | 223 | 230 | 236 | 243 |
| 70 | 132 | 139 | 146 | 153 | 160 | 167 | 174 | 181 | 188 | 195 | 202 | 209 | 216 | 222 | 229 | 236 | 243 | 250 |
| 71 | 136 | 143 | 150 | 157 | 165 | 172 | 179 | 186 | 193 | 200 | 208 | 215 | 222 | 229 | 236 | 243 | 250 | 257 |
| 72 | 140 | 147 | 154 | 162 | 169 | 177 | 184 | 191 | 199 | 206 | 213 | 221 | 228 | 235 | 242 | 250 | 258 | 265 |
| 73 | 144 | 151 | 159 | 166 | 174 | 182 | 189 | 197 | 204 | 212 | 219 | 227 | 235 | 242 | 250 | 257 | 265 | 272 |
| 74 | 148 | 155 | 163 | 171 | 179 | 186 | 194 | 202 | 210 | 218 | 225 | 233 | 241 | 249 | 256 | 264 | 272 | 280 |
| 75 | 152 | 160 | 168 | 176 | 184 | 192 | 200 | 208 | 216 | 224 | 232 | 240 | 248 | 256 | 264 | 272 | 279 | 287 |
| 76 | 156 | 164 | 172 | 180 | 189 | 197 | 205 | 213 | 221 | 230 | 238 | 246 | 254 | 263 | 271 | 279 | 287 | 295 |

| BMI | Obese | | | Extreme Obesity | | | | | | | | | | | | | | |
|---|---|---|---|---|---|---|---|---|---|---|---|---|---|---|---|---|---|---|
| | 37 | 38 | 39 | 40 | 41 | 42 | 43 | 44 | 45 | 46 | 47 | 48 | 49 | 50 | 51 | 52 | 53 | 54 |
| Height (inches) | Body Weight (pounds) | | | | | | | | | | | | | | | | | |
| 58 | 177 | 181 | 186 | 191 | 196 | 201 | 205 | 210 | 215 | 220 | 224 | 229 | 234 | 239 | 244 | 248 | 253 | 258 |
| 59 | 183 | 188 | 193 | 198 | 203 | 208 | 212 | 217 | 222 | 227 | 232 | 237 | 242 | 247 | 252 | 257 | 262 | 267 |
| 60 | 189 | 194 | 199 | 204 | 209 | 215 | 220 | 225 | 230 | 235 | 240 | 245 | 250 | 255 | 261 | 266 | 271 | 276 |
| 61 | 195 | 201 | 206 | 211 | 217 | 222 | 227 | 232 | 238 | 243 | 248 | 254 | 259 | 264 | 269 | 275 | 280 | 285 |
| 62 | 202 | 207 | 213 | 218 | 224 | 229 | 235 | 240 | 246 | 251 | 256 | 262 | 267 | 273 | 278 | 284 | 289 | 295 |
| 63 | 208 | 214 | 220 | 225 | 231 | 237 | 242 | 248 | 254 | 259 | 265 | 270 | 278 | 282 | 287 | 293 | 299 | 304 |
| 64 | 215 | 221 | 227 | 232 | 238 | 244 | 250 | 256 | 262 | 267 | 273 | 279 | 285 | 291 | 296 | 302 | 308 | 314 |
| 65 | 222 | 228 | 234 | 240 | 246 | 252 | 258 | 264 | 270 | 276 | 282 | 288 | 294 | 300 | 306 | 312 | 318 | 324 |
| 66 | 229 | 235 | 241 | 247 | 253 | 260 | 266 | 272 | 278 | 284 | 291 | 297 | 303 | 309 | 315 | 322 | 328 | 334 |
| 67 | 236 | 242 | 249 | 255 | 261 | 268 | 274 | 280 | 287 | 293 | 299 | 306 | 312 | 319 | 325 | 331 | 338 | 344 |
| 68 | 243 | 249 | 256 | 262 | 269 | 276 | 282 | 289 | 295 | 302 | 308 | 315 | 322 | 328 | 335 | 341 | 348 | 354 |
| 69 | 250 | 257 | 263 | 270 | 277 | 284 | 291 | 297 | 304 | 311 | 318 | 324 | 331 | 338 | 345 | 351 | 358 | 365 |
| 70 | 257 | 264 | 271 | 278 | 285 | 292 | 299 | 306 | 313 | 320 | 327 | 334 | 341 | 348 | 355 | 362 | 369 | 376 |
| 71 | 265 | 272 | 279 | 286 | 293 | 301 | 308 | 315 | 322 | 329 | 338 | 343 | 351 | 358 | 365 | 372 | 379 | 386 |
| 72 | 272 | 279 | 287 | 294 | 302 | 309 | 316 | 324 | 331 | 338 | 346 | 353 | 361 | 368 | 375 | 383 | 390 | 397 |
| 73 | 280 | 288 | 295 | 302 | 310 | 318 | 325 | 333 | 340 | 348 | 355 | 363 | 371 | 378 | 386 | 393 | 401 | 408 |
| 74 | 287 | 295 | 303 | 311 | 319 | 326 | 334 | 342 | 350 | 358 | 365 | 373 | 381 | 389 | 396 | 404 | 412 | 420 |
| 75 | 295 | 303 | 311 | 319 | 327 | 335 | 343 | 351 | 359 | 367 | 375 | 383 | 391 | 399 | 407 | 415 | 423 | 431 |
| 76 | 304 | 312 | 320 | 328 | 336 | 344 | 353 | 361 | 369 | 377 | 385 | 394 | 402 | 410 | 418 | 426 | 435 | 443 |

*Source:* Adapted from *Clinical Guidelines on the Identification, Evaluation, and Treatment of Overweight and Obesity in Adults: The Evidence Report* (National Institutes of Health, September 1998).

# Web Resources

National Heart, Lung, and Blood Institute   www.nhlbi.nih.gov

Weight-Control Information Network   www.win.niddk.gov

American Dietetic Association   www.eatright.org

American Diabetes Association   www.diabetes.org

NIH Office of Dietary Supplements   www.ods.od.nih.gov

American Heart Association   www.AmericanHeart.org

International Food Information Council (IFIC)   www.ific.org

American Institute for Cancer Research   www.aicr.org

American College of Sports Medicine   www.acsm.org

National Sleep Foundation   www.sleepfoundation.org

Mental Health America   www.nmha.org

American Society of Bariatric Physicians   www.asbp.org

American Society for Metabolic and Bariatric Surgery   www.asmbs.org

American Society of Plastic Surgeons   www.plasticsurgery.org

American Society for Aesthetic Plastic Surgery   www.surgery.org

# The Real You Tools

Here is a list of the basic tools from the four-point foundation of your BEAM Box, plus Power Tools, for your quick reference.

**Behavioral Tools**

(See chapter 3: Breaking Those Barriers to Success)
- Know and accept your eating style.
- Learn to change a habit.
- Identify reasons for emotional eating.
- Incorporate one change at a time.
- Use food to help manage emotional stress.
- Recognize "trigger" foods and avoid them.
- Reward yourself without using food.
- Address your life-coping skills.
- Weigh yourself regularly.
- Stay connected to your plan.
- Think before you drink or eat anything.
- Eat a morning meal.
- Aim for Level 2 of fullness.
- Minimize mindless eating.
- Agree there are no bad foods, just bad portions.
- Learn to barter.

- Keep your mouth busy with nonfood activities.
- Buy single servings.
- Accept your temperament.
- Commit to getting enough sleep.
- Remind yourself that daily activity is important.
- Wear a pedometer.
- Don't beat yourself up—learn from your mistakes.

## Eating/Food Tools

(See chapter 4: Choosing What to Eat)
- Bite and write: lifestyle logging.
- Read food labels.
- Choose "reverse calorie counting."
- Be a structured eater.
- Identify your eating temperament.
- Know your eating style.
- Avoid portion distortion.
- Choose how often to eat.
- Focus on foods that keep you full.
- Learn food bartering and exchanges.
- Choose lean proteins.
- Choose fruits and vegetables.
- Choose fiber-rich starches.
- Choose smart fats.
- Develop a Plan B.
- Be a positive snacker.
- Master restaurant eating.
- Get control of special occasion eating.
- Manage liquid calories and alcohol.
- Meet your vitamin and mineral needs.

## Activity Tools

(See chapter 5: How and When to Move)
- Know your physical activity temperament.
- Get started.

- Purchase a pedometer.
- Embrace the activity pyramid.
- Pace yourself: rate of perceived exertion.
- Focus on activity of daily living: move more every day.
- Pick up the pace with aerobic activity.
- Think about strength training.
- Strengthen your body core.
- Consider interval training.
- Stretch for better health.
- Consider mind-body activities.

## Medical/Biological Tools

(See chapter 6: Addressing Your Health Issues)
- How to talk to your doctor about your weight.
- Identify your weight-related risk factors.
- Identify your biological barriers to weight loss.
- Know your bloodwork "numbers."
- Size yourself up—connecting weight and health risk.
- Consider talking to your doctor about "power tools."
- Know about dietary supplements and nonprescription medications.

## Power Tools

(See chapter 8: Weight-Loss Medications and Surgery, and chapter 9: Body Contouring)
- Consider prescription medications.
- Consider obesity surgery options.
- Consider body contouring—what to do with hanging skin.

# Index